Eight Sure Steps to Health and Happiness

by Lucile H. Jones

REVIEW AND HERALD® PUBLISHING ASSOCIATION
Hagerstown, MD 21740

R & H Cataloging Service

Jones, Lucile Hall, 1910-
 Eight sure steps to health

 1. Health. 2. Self-care, Health.
I. Title.
 613
ISBN 0-8280-0468-4

CONTENTS

DEDICATED

To my parents, Charles and Lena Hall,
who first tossed out these lifesavers to me.

ACKNOWLEDGMENTS

Many very knowledgeable authorities have contributed to this book.

I am especially grateful to a number of most helpful acquaintances on the faculty of Loma Linda University.

In the University's School of Public Health, these include James Blankenship, Ph.D., professor of nutrition; Mervyn Hardinge, M.D., emeritus professor of health education; Patricia K. Johnston, D.P.H., director of the Doctor of Public Health Program; David C. Nieman, D.H.Sc., director of Health Science Program; Richard Neil, M.D., assistant dean; U. D. Register, Ph.D., emeritus professor of nutrition and dietetics; and Karen Burke, director of the Educational Materials Center.

Additionally, I wish to thank the following persons from the Loma Linda University School of Allied Health Professions: Lee Berk, D.H.Sc., associate professor of medical technology; Kenneth Burke, Ph.D., chairman of the Department of Nutrition and Dietetics; Georgia Hodgkin, M.Sc., assistant professor of nutrition and dietetics; Helen Seibert, M.Sc., assistant professor of physical therapy.

Other professionals who have shared their knowledge include Charles Thomas, D.P.H., of the Banning Preventive Health Care and Educational Center, Banning, California; Greg Goodchild, M.Sc., M.F.C.C., director of the Alcohol Recovery Program, Loma Linda Center for Health Promotion; Ralph Steinman, D.D.S., emeritus professor of dentistry, School of Dentistry, Loma Linda University; and Carl T. Jones, Ph.D., emeritus professor of chemistry, Walla Walla College.

Finally, Carol Ann Marlow, M.P.H., director of health education at Memorial Hospital in Manchester, Kentucky, contributed the "Lifesavers" theme of this book. I especially appreciate her help.

SUNSHINE

I glanced at the clock. "Right on time," I noted as I picked up our baby, freshly bathed and fed. I gave him another kiss, cuddled him in my arms, and carried him to his room while dreams of a bright future for him filled my mind. Snuggled in his warm crib, he took one deep breath, relaxed, and closed his sleepy eyes.

I checked a mental schedule—time to wash the dishes, put in a load of wash, make our bed, and iron a few pieces before my husband, Carl, would be home for lunch.

"I'll have to hurry," I told myself, "to get everything done and Jackie fed again before I leave for the three-to-eleven shift. A nurse's life certainly is full."

But my feet stopped still as I passed the living room window. "Now how does that girl do it?" I puzzled, watching my friend Terri Lynn briskly pushing her little Jimmie in his stroller. She looked so happy out there in the warm sunshine, a soft breeze ruffling her blonde hair, her eyes feasting on my neighbor's rose garden. Just for a moment I envied her.

Then I mused, "I bet her dishes aren't washed or her bed made. I wonder if she's ever gotten around to cleaning off those finger smudges I saw on her cupboard doors last week.

"Now, if we have to sacrifice a stroll in the sun and other leisurely pleasures to give our son a good home in this suburb, make car payments, and put away a little for his education, that's what we're going to do. He deserves the best."

I shrugged and turned away from the window, back to my unmade bed and dirty dishes. But my mind kept racing ahead of my hands. Were we really giving Jackie our best? Could Terri Lynn and little Jimmie be getting something that our baby was missing?

Could taking a walk outside in the fresh air and sunshine give Terri Lynn greater

calmness, cheerfulness, and strength to cope than I had? I had to admit some days were a bit hectic, and my anxious thoughts, hasty words, and feverish activities seemed to spill over onto my patient husband and crying baby.

For a number of weeks I continued this tightly scheduled rat race. Finally, one evening when I had the night off, I picked up a book, *The Ministry of Healing,* and started to read. The more I read, the more a calmness seemed to settle over me. I began to see how I could do better by my family.

> Pure air, sunlight, abstemiousness, rest, exercise, proper diet, the use of water, trust in divine power —these are the true remedies (p. 127).

My mind grasped the great truth—If these natural agents heal the sick, might they also improve our present quality of health?

Carl encouraged me as we worked out a plan. I scrutinized my daily activities and found I really could make some changes for the sake of my family.

I sandwiched in time to take Jackie outside while I planted tulip bulbs to bloom in the spring and to brighten our spirits as well as our yard.

We cut down and disposed of 21 pine trees from our backyard, letting in more sunlight to the baby's room and our kitchen and dining area. We put up an outdoor clothesline. (Don't you just love the smell of clean sheets dried in the sun and fresh air?)

Every afternoon at 2:15 I bundled my baby warmly, put on my uniform and cape, and stepped out into the beautiful autumn scen-

ery. Then I pushed the stroller over to my husband's office at the college just across campus from the hospital where I reported for work. At 5:00 he and the baby returned home for supper and an evening of fun together.

Soon we saw Jackie's eyes brighten, his cheeks grow rosy, and his energies bound. When the snows fell, we bundled him in a warm winter suit and took time out of our hectic lives to go sledding. We pulled him and the sled up the hill, then carefully sat beside him for a flying trip down the hill. Up and down we went, and Jackie laughed so hard that we forgot all our problems and projects.

By now these healthful activities held high priority in our home. We planned everything else around them.

When spring came and the sun again sprinkled freckles on my nose, I remembered my happy childhood in Florida. Sunshine always made me feel like singing, and by the time Jackie turned 2 years old, he could sing more than 20 happy choruses with me.

Our second child arrived to the warmth and sounds of a cheery home. Outside, a rose garden bordered with sweet alyssum welcomed him. A sandbox, slide, and a little black-and-white puppy coaxed him into an exciting outdoor life. At the hospital I worked faithfully and prayed that God would bless my efforts to apply His healing agents to my hurting patients.

"But how much better it would be," I kept telling myself, "if I could keep them from getting sick." So when another college called Carl and offered to sponsor him for a graduate program, I grabbed the opportunity to register for courses in which I could learn more about these lifesavers—sunshine, fresh air, abstemiousness, rest, exercise, proper diet, water, and trust in divine power.

While we studied we lived in a small apartment and pinched our few pennies to make ends meet. Nevertheless, we managed to buy four tennis rackets and a few balls, and with our boys, reveled in the sunshine and fresh air that rested and energized our tired brains.

Some people say that sunshine acts like a tranquilizer, but for me it's more often a stimulator. It makes my spirits soar.

Sunlight appears to help many travelers overcome the effects of jetlag. Walking about in the sunlight after a nightflight will relieve feelings of tiredness and make you more alert.

I studied not only for grades but to learn how to help people keep well. I devoured my lessons and library assignments, grateful for the opportunity to learn more about God's lifesavers for us.

I learned that our wise Creator made sunlight to bring a wealth of beauty into our lives. Not only does sunshine make our flowers grow, but it adds green chlorophyll to the leaves and color to the blossoms. What a dull world this would be without red roses, yellow daffodils, and pink petunias.

Sunshine also heats the volatile oils in flowers and fruit and scatters their perfume—rich and fragrant—through air currents set in motion by the sun's rays.

In ripening fruit the sunshine changes starch to sugar to sweeten strawberries, cherries, and oranges. Yet that very same light ripens the corn, wheat, and oats by turning sugar to starch.

In springtime the sun melts the snow to fill our lakes and rivers with life-renewing water. It awakens hibernating animals and triggers the nesting hormone in birds.

Yet all of this is but a fraction of what God does for you and me through the sun, which is located some 93 million miles away. Sunlight truly is a lifesaver. It builds vitamin D in your skin, enabling you to use calcium, which is necessary for building strong bones and teeth.

I never will forget the day our little neighbor, Cindy, jumped on her horse and galloped across the pasture. But the pony made an unexpected turn, and Cindy flew off, hitting the ground with a thud. She tried to get up, but with two broken arms she had to turn and twist, get on her knees, and finally to her feet. With her two floppy arms held closely to her chest and with tears dripping from her cheeks, she walked back to the gate and her horrified mother. What could Cindy do to help her bones heal fast? Get plenty of sunshine, of course—and that's just what she did.

Ralph Steinman, D.D.S., of Yucaipa, California, agrees that sunshine makes a difference in your teeth, too. He says, "In the service I did dental work on men in many areas overseas. We observed that those from

Iceland and areas where the skies are cloudy had much worse dental decay than those who had spent their time in the tropics, where the sun beat down on them many hours a day." He went on to say that he found the same comparison to be true in the States. The teeth of those he treated from New England were in worse condition than those from Texas, New Mexico, and California, where sunshine is more abundant. [1]

Sunshine also increases the activity of your liver. This means that with additional light, premature babies with skin yellowed by jaundice can rapidly recover before the condition damages their brains or causes death.

The infrared (heat) rays of sunlight penetrate deeply into the body, aiding the circulatory and muscle systems.

To guard your health, the sun kills germs all around you. Dr. Lawrence P. Garrod, professor of bacteriology at the University of London, found that the dust under the bed and in the dark corners of hospital rooms was loaded with disease-producing bacteria, but dust from near the window or on the windowsill had much less. He says that ordinary daylight, even on a cloudy day in winter, does kill bacteria.

Not only does sunshine kill germs all around you, but it also increases the number of white cells your body produces to fight and destroy germs that manage to get inside your body.

You need to take a few precautions when getting out in the sun. While a little sunshine is good, a lot is not.

In winter a good time to get outside is between 10:00 in the morning and noon. In summer it's better to get out early, around 8:30 or 9:00, before the sun is too hot.

Not only does sunburn make you uncomfortable, but too much sunshine can even encourage cancer growth.

Without light we see no color. Everything is in shades of gray and black. But in the sunshine everything quickly comes to life, for light brings out the beauty of color.

Color affects you more than you realize. It affects your personality and mental outlook. Each color bring its own beautiful memories.

The bright yellow of sunshine brings cheer and makes you feel warm.

> Yellow is butterflies bathed in light,
> A field of daisies and daffodils bright.
> It's corn bread and butter, a pot of honey,
> A candle's flicker, a day that is sunny. [2]

Red makes you more alert and active.

> Red is a fire engine, bright and exciting.
> Or a pale pink rose with petals inviting.
> It's a ripe tomato plucked from the vine,
> Or candy cotton from some early time.
> It's a hunter's coat, a tartan clan,
> A satin ribbon, a peppermint band.
> It's strawberries, melon, and good things
>   to eat.
> Red is exciting and always a treat. [3]

Orange is another warm and lovely color.

Orange is a flame mixed with emotion.
It's a painted sunset across the ocean.
It's the color of autumn, rich in appeal,
Nutmeg and pumpkins, a Thanksgiving
    meal.
Burnt or bittersweet, peachy or bright,
Orange as an accent can be just right.[4]

The cool colors—blue, green, and blue-green—found in the sky, the trees, and grasses are calming and relaxing. This is another reason that walking outdoors is such a health-promoting practice.

Blue is the sky on a bright summer day,
Or it's cold and bleak in a winter way.
Blue is the sea, a fish, or a book,
An aster, a sapphire, a feeling, a look.
It's a blue-winged teal that quacks aloud.
Blue is majesty wrapped in a cloud.[5]

Green has universal appeal. It is the most restful of all colors. It is the principal color in nature, providing a rich background for all other colors.

Green is the springtime after the snow
Rich and appealing, Nature's aglow.
It's a doorway at Christmas, an emerald
    ball,
The ocean in summer, an evergreen tall.
Green is a cucumber, a salad that's crisp.
Green as a color is never a risk.[6]

To start your day off right, why not get up early enough tomorrow morning to watch the sun peek over the eastern horizon to greet the world with glorious color, boundless energy, and healing rays?

---

[1] Interview with Ralph Steinman, D.D.S., Yucaipa, California, Dec. 22, 1987.
[2] "Come Catch a Rainbow" (PPG Industries, 1967), p. 2.
[3] *Ibid.*, p. 6.
[4] *Ibid.*, p. 8.
[5] *Ibid.*, p. 4.
[6] *Ibid.*, p. 10.

Lifesaver 2

FRESH AIR

We stretched on tiptoe to catch the last golden glow of a lovely sunset, then turned to the warmth of our campfire in the Blue Mountains of northeastern Oregon.

Silently we sat for a few moments, lost in memories and dreams that such scenes inspire. Then someone asked, "What's the most beautiful sound you've ever enjoyed?"

We looked at one another, at the shadowy hillsides, and reminisced of the past several decades. A smile crept across the face of a dedicated bird-watcher. "I think there is nothing more beautiful than the sound of happy birds."

What memories this brought of the Southland where the mockingbird sings and the cardinal whistles his elegant call; memories of brightly colored squawking parrots and birds in the Far East with strange songs; memories of an early-morning strawberry patch in Washington State, where the meadowlarks serenaded as we gathered berries for the freezer.

A World War II veteran recalled the delicate sound of tinkling cowbells in the peaceful pastures of Switzerland.

Others thought of soothing sounds of waterfalls, rippling streams, lapping waves on a sandy beach, or even the whistling of a tea-kettle in a happy home.

Another thought of a person lost on a rugged mountain and the sound of H-O-P-E spelled by the throb of a helicopter.

I remembered another sound dear to me as a child. I can almost hear it now—the horn of my father's car as it turned into our driveway.

A young mother thought of the welcome cry of her newborn; and a grandfather, with his arm about his white-haired wife, declared, "I think the most beautiful thing I remember is the 'I do' spoken by my bride 40 years ago."

Perhaps among the most welcome words to any mother's ear are "Hi, Mom!" I prick up my ears and my heart skips a beat when I hear an amateur radio operator saying

"WA7YBA, WA7YBA, WA7YBA. This is WA6GPO calling on schedule and standing by." That's our son—calling home from 1200 miles away.

To others, beauty means the sound of inspiring music, the only language in which you cannot say a mean or sarcastic thing. The person who has a song in his heart as well as on his lips is well armored against the drab assaults of life. There is more than beauty in song; there is strength and courage.

> And the Lord God formed man of the dust of the ground, and breathed into his nostrils the breath of life; and man became a living soul (Genesis 2:7).

What a marvelous medium is air! Although sound travels through water and other media, the air is all around us and carries the sounds right into our ears, where it sets the "keyboard" of the inner ear vibrating so that we can hear beautiful, exciting, sad, or warning messages.

Regardless of the health and size of your vocal cords, you couldn't talk or sing if you exhaled no air from your lungs to set them vibrating.

When oxygen in the air combines with your food, it supplies energy for your brain to think, your heart to beat, and for your muscles to contract so you can walk, bend, reach, sit, or lie down.

When you work hard or play hard, when you jog or run, you get very warm. How do you cool off again? One good way is simply to let the air evaporate the perspiration on your skin.

When a member of your family is sick and has a high fever, you can bring his temperature down and make him much more comfortable by smoothing a little moisture (either water or rubbing alcohol) on his skin. Apply it to only one arm, leg, or other part at a time so he won't become chilled. Then fan it gently and slowly with your hand. As the air evaporates the moisture, it cools. In this way it is an effective aid in temperature control.

Full, deep breaths of pure air get more oxygen down deep into the lower clusters of air sacs of your lungs. This helps to clear out the germs that collect down there and might start disease.

Fresh air speeds up the circulation of your blood, getting more oxygen and nutrition to all your cells, and better removing wastes so you can think and work efficiently.

When you're sick, fresh air and sunshine can help you to get well sooner. The sunshine lifts your spirits and gives a calmness that puts your mind at ease, while both sunshine and fresh air kill germs.

For this reason, before we had modern medications, resting or sleeping outdoors was one of the earliest treatments for patients with tuberculosis.

Fresh air helps to calm your nerves and enables you to sleep more soundly. Perhaps this is one reason so many young families today enjoy hiking and camping on weekends and vacations. Others are moving their families to the country, where the air is freer of pollutants.

If you are a shallow breather, you limit the amount of oxygen you take in to keep your brain alert, and you may be missing the lift you could have to chase away depression.

To help me remember to breathe deeply, I

put a little reminder sign, "Breathe Deeply," on my bathroom mirror and on the upper part of my stove in the kitchen.

In your home you will want to avoid too much humidity in the air. In summer it can make you feel hotter, sticky, uncomfortable, and even depressed. In winter it will make you feel chilly. You can guard against this by not letting a teakettle or a coffee maker steam unnecessarily in your kitchen. You may want to shorten your hot showers to prevent getting excess moisture into the air.

However, if the air is too dry, your throat may become irritated. The little cilia (hairlike projections) in your air passages don't wave the germs up and out, as they normally do.

T he ingredients of health and long life, are great temperance, open air, easy labor, and little care."

Sir Philip Sidney

Overexposure to cold air is dangerous because your blood pressure is raised in an endeavor to keep you warm. This puts an extra load on your heart. When you feel cold, there are fewer active white cells in your blood stream. Remember, they are your germ fighters, your lifesavers, so when they are not in there ready to attack the germs, your resistance to colds and other infections is lowered.

You probably have noticed that air that is too warm makes you feel tired more quickly.

You can't get as much done as you normally do. This is why you need air within the proper temperature (60 to 80 degrees) and humidity range (30 to 65 percent).

One of our big problems today is air pollution. Every year industrial plants and cars spew out millions of tons of air contaminants—solid particles, gases, and liquid droplets. When we add to this the dust, pollens, insecticides, and smoke in a stagnant air pocket, we have a disease-producing atmosphere.

During the day plants and trees take in carbon dioxide and give off oxygen. We and other animals take oxygen from the air and return carbon dioxide to it. This is the balance God planned for us when He placed Adam and Eve in a garden home. But we have cut down our forests and built factories and cars to contaminate our atmosphere.

During periods of dense smog in large cities the death rates rise. That is why we have smog alerts over the radio and TV warning us, especially the aged or ill, to stay inside and use our air conditioners.

If you decide to get a good air conditioning unit that not only recirculates the air but brings in fresh air and filters it, you may find it well worth the cost in terms of your family's health.

So when the air is clear, it is worth a lot to your family's health to see that all get outside to breathe deeply and enjoy its lifesaving benefits.

If you have added storm windows and weather stripping to keep your house warm and cozy during the winter months, you may cut your heating bills. However, you will want to take precautions to make sure that

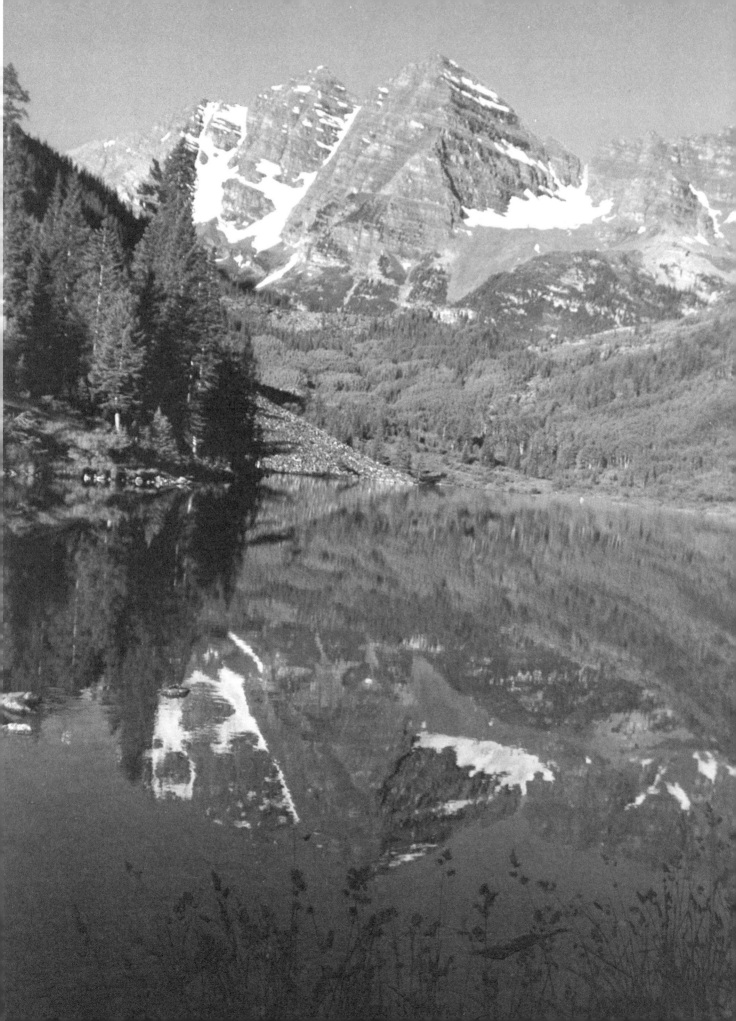

you don't use any open flames in a gas stove, furnace, or heater without good ventilation, because of the poisonous carbon monoxide that they may produce.

If you notice that you develop a headache, feel weak and tired, and have a problem sleeping well over the weekend, then feel much better when you go back to work the first of the week, you might do well to check your ventilation system.

The School of Public Health at the University of California at Berkeley gives several good suggestions for keeping the air in your home safe. Even if you don't sense any problems, it still is worth taking these precautions:

"1. Have a reputable heating company inspect your furnace, the flue, and the vent connector pipe. Replace any rusted or damaged parts. If converting from one type of fuel to another, it is best to get a qualified technician to do the work.

2. Make sure your gas range has an exhaust fan vented to the outside. Use the fan every time you cook.

3. Vent all fuel-burning heaters to the outside. Don't take a chance.

4. Never use a gas range or oven to heat a room, even during a power outage.

5. Don't leave a pot of water boiling on a gas flame all day to boost humidity. Instead, just set a pan of water on the radiator, or use a humidifier.

6. Setting up the hibachi in the house may sound like fun, but burning charcoal may generate carbon monoxide. Even in a fireplace, fumes may back up into the room." [1]

If you have a cool-air humidifier, it is a good practice to wash the water container every time you use it. Bacteria and molds thrive in damp places, and when you turn the humidifier on again, it may spray these into the air to cause allergic reactions and lung infections. Ultrasonic humidifiers do kill bacteria and molds, but you still will want to clean the humidifier at least once a week. [2]

Although oxygen and sunshine in the air are germ killers, this does not mean they purify the air of the poisons present in smog and tobacco smoke.

Without realizing it, you can be laying the foundation for cancer in your spouse and children. If you smoke in your home, you make your family become passive (secondhand) smokers. They breathe in the many poisons that are contained in tobacco smoke. These include carbon monoxide and cancer-related nicotine. T. Hirayama, M.D., of the National Cancer Center Research Institute, affirms this in his study of families in Japan. He says: "Up to twofold increase in mortality from lung cancer was observed in the nonsmoking wives of husbands who smoked. The effects of passive smoking was found to be one half to one third that of direct smoking in terms of relative risk of lung cancer." [3]

Apparently, the more you or your family inhale tobacco smoke, whether at home, at work, or in other contacts, the greater is your (and their) risk of developing lung cancer.

Shigeru Matsukura, M.D., and his associates report in the *New England Journal of Medicine* the conclusions of their study of passive smokers: "We conclude that the deleterious effects of passive smoking may occur in proportion to the exposure of nonsmokers to smokers in the home, the workplace, and the community." [4] This shows us the effects of tobacco smoking anywhere can be dangerous to your health—even if you are a nonsmoker.

A woman who is really interested in the best health for her baby will not smoke during pregnancy, she will not smoke during lactation, and she will not smoke while she is raising her child. [5]

Do you think the effect of your exhaled poisons is only temporary? Tomorrow it won't make any difference? Or tomorrow you will stop smoking and all will be well? Listen to what Ann Charlton reports in a recent *British Medical Journal.* She says: "Results are clear evidence of a definite link between smoking in the home and coughs in young children, which not only may present immediate problems but may also be a cause of illness in the future." [6]

Regardless of the fact that we have really messed up our atmosphere terribly, there still are many blessings that it brings to us. For instance, air pressure enables the insects, birds, and planes to fly. Its buoyancy makes balloons rise.

We also enjoy the cushioning effect of air in such things as tires, pillows, and air mattresses.

Air is a natural transportation system for moisture, seeds, pollens, and odors. It transmits sound. It is by means of these odors in the air that insects find their homes, their food, and their mates. And that's how mosquitoes can find you, even in the dark!

But on the brighter side, can't we be thankful for the scents of fresh apples, opening roses, a sprig of mint, and freshly baked bread?

"Wind," a little boy once explained, "is air in a hurry."

One of the nice things about "air in a hurry" is that it turns the windmills to pump water and do other tasks. It also makes our sailboats skim gracefully over the water and colorful kites to fly high in the sky.

Now can you better appreciate God's great wisdom in giving us air on the second day of Creation? He had it all ready and waiting for the fragrance of the flowers on the third day, the song of the birds on the fifth, the sense of smell for the animals on the sixth, and ready for Eve to hear Adam say "I love you" that Friday afternoon.

---

[1] *Berkeley Wellness Letter,* January 1988, p. 7.

[2] *Ibid.,* p. 1.

[3] *British Medical Journal* 282 (1981): 183-185.

[4] *New England Journal of Medicine* 311 (1984): 828-832.

[5] C. Everett Koop, surgeon general of the United States, in *Vibrant Life,* December 1985, pp. 17-19, 47.

[6] Anne Charlton, in *British Medical Journal* 288 (1984): .

ABSTEMIOUSNESS

(TEMPERANCE)

Poor Jake Jenkins! I pitied my neighbor, lying there so depressed and discouraged, his right foot propped up on two pillows. He looked pale, and his weak voice made me fear he had but a few days left to live. A faint moan escaped his tight lips as he tried to move his foot to a slightly different position.

His frail little wife looked so worn that I asked what I might do to help her.

"I'm not very good at giving a bath to anybody in bed," she said. "And I'm so afraid of hurting his bad foot. Would you have time to help me with that?"

Glad to have one last chance to do something for him and to help Mrs. Jenkins, I gently washed and dried him, changed the sheets, and adjusted his leg to a more comfortable position.

As we stepped outside the house I asked Mrs. Jenkins, "What's the matter with Jake's foot? Did infection set in after some injury?"

"No." She looked down as if she hated to admit the cause. "It came on gradually, over the past six months. The doctor says it's Buerger's disease."

Right away I knew why his right foot was so discolored. In fact, it looked as if it was dead. Buerger's disease is caused by the poisons in tobacco smoke. It is an inflammation and clogging of the tiny blood vessels, cutting off the blood supply and resulting in gangrene of the fingers and toes.

Jake had only one chance to extend his life—surgery to remove his leg. He didn't want to go to the hospital—but he didn't want to die, either. He was not an old man. He wanted to see Bill, his son, become a successful businessman. He wanted to live to help his weary wife. They both wanted to live to enjoy their grandchildren. But Jake had just two grim choices—die within weeks, with two legs, or possibly live a little longer

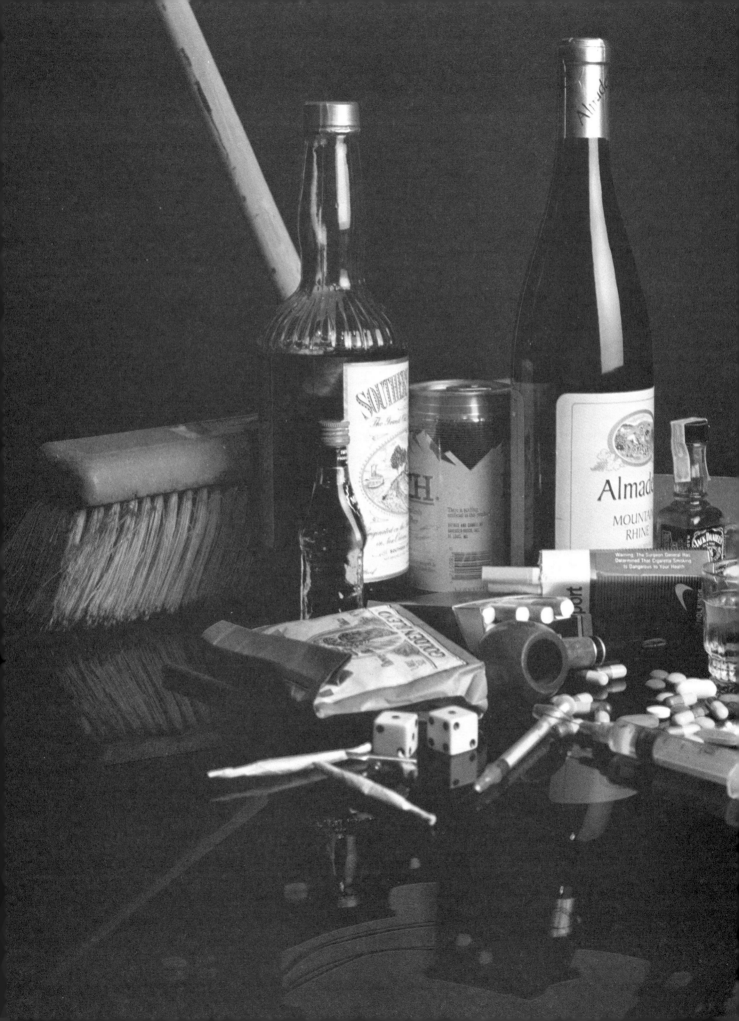

with only a left leg—if he was willing to throw away his cigarettes.

A second opinion gave no more hope, so he chose surgery. Bill, seeing that smoking had cheated his dad not only of health but of his very life, promised, "I'm quitting too. No more tobacco for me."

Although Jake Jenkins survived a few months, the damage done to him was not confined to his black toes and purple foot.

Soon his heart, seriously affected by the poisons in tobacco smoke, gave out, leaving Mrs. Jenkins to struggle on alone.

Bill had good intentions, and I probably never would have remembered this family except for one sad incident.

Walking to the post office one day, I thought I saw Bill coming toward me. I blinked and looked again. Could it really be Bill—puffing on a cigarette?

While still about half a block away, Bill looked up and saw me. He promptly jaywalked across the street and passed by with his head turned the other way.

Bill is typical of young people addicted to tobacco smoking.

It fastens them so tightly in its grip that without special help they find it impossible to shake the habit.

Irritating particles in cigarette smoke cause a constriction of the small air tubes in your lungs. Some of the poisons also paralyze or slow down the waving motion of the little cilia in the air passages. Then they can't bring up mucus and waste particles from the depths of the lungs to the throat, where they can be coughed up and spit out. When they cannot do their work, germs and other irritants collect deep in the lungs and may pave the way for such problems as emphysema or lung cancer.

Tobacco smoke also affects your heart. It makes it beat faster and increases your blood pressure. It causes irregularities in the rhythm of your heartbeat and constricts the blood vessels of your skin. This is why smokers often have cold feet and hands and sallow faces.

All of this adds to the work of your heart; and if you smoke, you greatly increase your risk of heart attacks.

Another risky practice you'll want to avoid is the use of "smokeless tobacco." Whether you chew it or just hold it in your mouth, it is extremely dangerous. It may lead to cancer of the mouth, gums, or throat. The sad part is that reports show that a surprising number of young people, including kindergarten children, are using "smokeless tobacco," without any understanding of the tragic risks it poses. [1]

> **Choose rather to punish your appetites than to be punished by them."**
> Tyrius Maximus

Experiments with both rabbits and people show that nicotine by mouth raises total cholesterol and LDL cholesterol (the harmful kind) and lowers HDL cholesterol (the helpful kind). The widespread use of smokeless tobacco and nicotine chewing gum makes these findings most important to us as parents. We need to warn our boys and girls, set a good example for them, and provide other peer-approved behavior. [2]

William L. Weis, Ph.D., professor of accounting at Seattle University, says, "Recent employee surveys taken within major American companies and government agencies show that between 70 and 80 percent of employees don't want to work around colleagues who smoke. . . . In a survey that I conducted with a colleague . . . involving 223 management personnel who were directly responsible for hiring their subordinates, 53.4 percent indicated that they chose nonsmokers over smokers when faced with similarly qualified job seekers. [3]

So whether you are a man or woman, you may improve your prospects of getting that special job if you choose not to smoke.

If you were an employer, wouldn't you prefer nonsmokers who are healthier, have higher morale, and miss fewer days from work?

If you are smart, you won't be misled by tobacco advertisements. The fact that smokers are being hired less often than nonsmokers is frightening the tobacco companies so much that they are trying to counteract the truths by picturing professional people at work with cigarettes either in their fingers or mouths.

Weis says the truth is getting around "that smoking is no longer an appropriate social behavior" in the professional world. "To a mature, responsible adult, smoker or nonsmoker, the spectacle of young people smoking looks stupid and immature—not sophisticated and grown-up." [4]

In an interview with Ralph Blodgett, former editor of *Vibrant Life,* Dr. C. Everett Koop, surgeon general of the United States, said that smoking is even more addictive than alcohol and that it is much harder for a smoker to give up his tobacco than it is for an alcoholic to leave off his drinking—and that's pretty hard. [5]

Many young people think they can stop smoking any time they choose, but when they decide to try it alone, they discover it is almost impossible.

First, you need God's help, and you need the help of some experienced successful program like the Five-Day Plan to Stop Smoking, sponsored by the Seventh-day Adventist Church.

J. Wayne McFarland, M.D., promoter of the Five-Day Plan, suggests some things that may make it easier for you to stop smoking.

He feels your best way is to stop all at once rather than cutting down slowly. The first three days will be your hardest, but every day without the tobacco poisons gives you a great feeling of accomplishment and self-respect. Remember, this is your own decision, so when the going gets rough you can keep telling yourself, "I choose not to smoke."

He says that when the craving hits, you should take a look at your watch. Every second you are able to keep your hand off a cigarette gives you courage to continue. When you have watched the second hand go all the way around and see you have succeeded for a whole minute, you think, *I did it for one minute. I can do that again. And again.* After only three minutes you probably will notice the craving is subsiding.

Here are other practices that can help you to stay away from tobacco:

1. Bathe frequently. This helps to remove the poisons and odor eliminated through the skin. To relieve intense craving

you may find a hot shower followed by a cold one most helpful.

2. Drink at least six glasses of water every day. Besides quenching your thirst, water dilutes the poisons and lightens the work of your kidneys.

3. Have a regular time for meals, sleep, and major activities, and stick to your schedule. This can help you to resist the craving.

4. Don't sit around after eating. Instead of relaxing in your favorite (tobacco-smelly) chair after meals, taking a good walk outside will give you better success in sticking to your decision.

5. Leave off all drinks that contain alcohol, caffeine, or other sedatives or stimulants. Substitute milk, buttermilk, or hot cereal drinks, which don't precipitate the craving .

6. Omit highly spiced foods, steaks, fried foods, rich foods, and those high in sugar.

7. Eat all you want of fruit, grains, vegetables, and a few nuts, but no snacks.

8. Breathe deeply and have good posture.

9. Take no tablets or other aids to help you stop smoking unless you check with your doctor first.

10. Trust in God to help you. He has limitless power. [6]

If you or a friend of yours would like help to kick the habit, contact your local Seventh-day Adventist church for information about its stop-smoking clinics.

The United States Department of Health and Human Services has published an excellent pamphlet, *Good for You, a Guide to Living as a Nonsmoker.* It recommends that when you have the urge to smoke, you stop and review your reasons for quitting. The following reasons are on most people's lists:

1. I want to set a good example for my children.
2. Smoking makes my clothes smell. My hair, too.
3. Smoking is bad for my health.
4. I want to get rid of my smoker's cough.
5. I don't want to be a slave to a bad habit. I want to be more in control of my life.
6. Smoking is a waste of money. I don't want to spend any more money on a bad habit.
7. Smoking around nonsmokers makes me feel uncomfortable. [7]

Are you afraid of gaining weight if you stop smoking? Before you go on a questionable diet, continue the practices listed above, starting with a substantial breakfast, a good noon meal, and little or no supper.

man ever repented that he arose from the table sober, healthful, and with his wits about him."

Jeremy Taylor

Art Thompson, a courteous, polite, but shy young man, needed friends. So when a couple of fellows who worked in the same printshop as he did, asked him to stop by the local bar with them after work one Friday afternoon, he smiled and said, "Sure. Why not?"

Something about the place, the people there, or the drinks made him feel at ease. Because of this, he began to stop by for a drink several times a week, and sometimes he took another along home for later that evening. Whiskey gradually became his companion. It helped him forget his problems and his loneliness in the big city of Allentown, Pennsylvania.

Art didn't realize what was happening to his health, his brain, his personality, and his future. He just turned more and more to drinking.

He didn't care about going to church anymore. He sometimes wished he had more money left from his weekly paycheck to buy a box of candy or beautiful flowers for his girlfriend, Margie. He loved her, and he could tell she really cared about him. Sometimes she ventured softly, "Artie, you'd be better off without that drink."

But she was too smart to nag, and she was too smart to smoke or drink. She just seemed to feel sorry for him. As the months slipped into years and their friendship grew, Art finally worked up enough courage to tell her, "Margie, I need you. I could never do without you. I'm 34 years old. It's time I got married. And there's nobody else but you. Couldn't we go the rest of the way together?"

He saw that wistful look in her sad eyes and felt her squeeze his hand—but then, just as he feared, she took a deep breath and spoke the words that shattered his dreams. "Art, I love you. But I hate alcohol. I will never marry that booze bottle. You will have to choose between me and alcohol."

"I'll try," he promised. "I can never give you up."

Art tried, but alcohol and tobacco had taken away his willpower.

He developed a hacking cough. He hated himself as much as he loved Margie. He thought he would do anything in the world to make her happy and to have her with him. But he had no strength to resist alcohol.

Wine is a mocker, strong drink is raging: and whosoever is deceived thereby is not wise (Proverbs 20:1).

Art lived on alone. And Margie, always hoping and wishing he would change, watched him grow thinner and weaker as the cigarette poisons and alcohol wrecked not only his body but his personality as well.

Art told himself over and over, "If only I could start over. I'd *never* take that first drink nor smoke that first cigarette.

One day as he watched his 4-year-old nephew playing happily and buoyantly, he called him aside, held him firmly, shook his finger in the boy's face and threatened, "Todd, if ever I find you smoking one cigarette, I'll beat the very daylights out of you." Todd ran away in fright; but Art had threatened not because he hated the child but because he loved Todd too much to think of tobacco and alcohol taking away his happiness, health, and life as it was doing to him.

Finally, as cancer ravaged Art's lungs and stomach, he realized it was too late—too late for a happy family, too late for a successful career, too late for life!

Poor Art! He must have felt like Robert McChesney did when he lay dying and confessed to his friend: "God gave me a horse and a message. Alas, I killed the horse, and now I cannot deliver the message."

Alcohol is a deceptive drug. It acts first upon the higher nerve centers in the front part of your brain, where you think and make judgments and decisions.[8] Here it also releases your inhibitions and gives you a false sense of superiority. As you drink more, alcohol depresses the nerve centers on the top and sides of your brain, benumbing your sensations and slowing your muscle activity. After this, it reaches the lower areas that control your breathing and heartbeat. When it paralyzes these, you are on your way out, for whatever gets your brain gets you! "There is no cure for alcoholism except abstinence."[9]

But it's not too late for you to take hold of the Power that can free you from the bonds of alcohol. Rein up your horse and "go for it."

An experiment which Dr. U. D. Register, chairman of the Department of Nutrition, Loma Linda University, did on rats suggests how the diet of typical American teenagers may help develop the taste for alcoholic beverages before they realize it.

He divided the rats into two groups. He fed one group on a poor diet, typical of many American teenagers. It consisted of two glazed doughnuts for breakfast; at 10:00 a sweet roll; a noon meal of a hotdog, a soft drink, and apple pie; at 3:00 p.m. another sweet roll; and at dinner, meatballs and spaghetti, two slices of garlic bread, green beans, tossed fresh vegetable salad, and chocolate cake. Then a TV snack of three filled cookies and a candy bar.

He fed the second group of rats a lacto-vegetarian diet. It was made up of milk, a vegetarian entrée, potatoes, vegetables, salad, bread, etc.

He gave each rat two water bottles, one containing plain water and one with 10 percent alcohol in water.

The rats on the poor diet more often chose the alcoholic drink, while those on the good diet chose the water. Evidently a poor diet increases the desire to drink alcoholic beverages.[10]

Why not help your children to build resistance to drinking alcoholic beverages by giving them a good, nutritious diet without coffee and spices?

God
will not work a miracle to keep those from sickness who have no care for themselves, but are continually violating the laws of health and make no efforts to prevent disease."
E. G. White

J. S. Gill and associates in their study found another danger of using alcohol. Their data show that heavy drinking of alcoholic beverages is an important, although unrecognized, risk factor for stroke in men. They discovered that heavy drinkers are four times as likely to have a stroke as those who do not drink.[11]

If you drink, you should, not only for your own sake but for that of your children, join the thousands who are breaking the drinking habit. Dr. Greg Goodchild, director of the Clearview Alcohol and Drug Dependency Program of the Loma Linda Community Hospital in Loma Linda, California, says that chemical dependency is transferred from parents to their children. He then introduced me to Craig Richards, a typical drug-dependent person, who told me his story.[12]

"My grandfather drank," he said. "And my mother has been an active drug abuser for more than 20 years. She doesn't even realize it because she takes only prescribed drugs, but she is addicted just the same.

"I grew up with a drug-dependent background, poor judgment, poor self-control, a lack of security and a distrust of adults.

"After my eighteenth birthday I joined the military, where I could easily get alcohol and cigarettes. I would take up to 20 cans of beer, plus other drugs, to my room at night. Then in Vietnam I added marijuana and began to listen to hard rock music.

"After I came back to the States, I was arrested for driving while drunk, so I decided that drinking and driving don't mix. Now could you guess what I did?"

He laughed. Just remember how important a driver's license is to a 20-year-old!

"Well, I was so dependent on drugs that I even gave up driving for several months.

"Alcohol and drugs are that important to an addict.

"But in spite of my background, my strong dependency, and the hold alcohol had on me, God reached me through several experiences, one of which seems unbelievable.

"While 'under the influence' one night, I actually drove a car 20 miles with the left front brake burned out. It melted the wheel mechanism down to the very axle. And when I got out and looked at it, I wondered why in the world that wheel hadn't fallen off.

"This really shook me up, and I began to think about my condition. I even began reading my Bible. God gave me the power to break the stronghold of alcohol and tobacco. From the time I prayed from a sincere heart, 'Lord, I have a problem, and I can't do a thing about it. I need You,' the craving for cigarettes and alcohol vanished. I followed through the 12 steps of the Alcoholics Anonymous program, and God gave me a new heart, new interests, and new goals."

Craig's little daughter, with three generations of drug addiction behind her, has an 80 percent risk of becoming drug-dependent, Dr. Goodchild told me. However, Craig is doing all he can to provide a good environment for her. He has gone back to school and with a professional preparation has dedicated his life to promoting God's plan of helping His drug-dependent children.

The Alcoholics Anonymous organization helps men and women who want to get away from alcohol. You can find it listed in your telephone book. Their buddy system and the following 12 steps to recovery can help you.

"1. We admitted we were powerless over alcohol—that our lives had become unmanageable.

"2. Came to believe that a power greater than ourselves could restore us to sanity.

"3. Made a decision to turn our will and our lives over to the care of God as we understood Him.

"4. Made a searching and fearless moral inventory of ourselves.

"5. Admitted to God, to ourselves, and to another human being the exact nature of our wrongs.

" 6. Were entirely ready to have God remove all these defects of character.

" 7. Humbly asked Him to remove our shortcomings.

" 8. Made a list of all persons we had harmed, and became willing to make amends to them all.

" 9. Made direct amends to such people wherever possible, except when to do so would injure them or others.

"10. Continued to take personal inventory and when we were wrong promptly admitted it.

"11. Sought through prayer and meditation to improve our conscious contact with God as we understood Him, praying only for knowledge of His will for us and the power to carry that out.

"12. Having had a spiritual awakening as the result of these steps, we tried to carry this message to alcoholics and to practice these principles in all our affairs."

The Alanon group is most helpful to spouses and children of alcoholics. It can help you to gain understanding, encouragement, and strength to cope with the problems of alcoholics and their families. And remember, God has all the answers. He too is waiting to help you.

But how much better it is to help prevent our young people from becoming dependent on drugs. Dr. Patricia Mutch, director of the Institute of Alcoholism and Drug Dependency, Andrews University, found in her study that "young people involved in certain types of religious experiences were less likely to show involvement with drugs."

"Among those who used drugs in the past, the use was dramatically less when youth had participated in:

"1. Family worship.

"2. Temperance contests.

"3. Telling someone else about their faith.

"Among those who presently used drugs, the use was dramatically less when youth were participating in:

"1. Family worship.

"2. Church-sponsored social events.

"3. Personal prayer." [13]

We should never look down on intemperate persons, for temperance is more than saying no to alcoholic drinks, pills, powders, and pop. It also means avoiding overwork, overeating, overexercising. It also includes avoiding such things as driving all night, reading very exciting books, or anything that drastically depletes your energy. It can include anything that builds up a high level of stress— things like worry.

I found this out one fateful morning. A seriously ill relative needed medication at once. I already had a packed schedule that day. But with my mind in a whirl, I ran to my car, drove quickly to the pharmacy, got the prescription refilled, and started back with it.

However, it happened that on that very morning a young friend of mine teetered on the verge of a tragic decision. I feared lest his choice would wreck his life. I could see that it might easily deprive him of future happiness, his church relationship, and possibly his chance for eternal life.

I had to pray about all these things. So while driving, I put my whole heart and soul into telling God a few things I thought He ought to do.

I thought I had my eyes open. But in my haste and worry, I didn't see the stop sign on my right, nor the car coming from my left. Wham! It hit hard! It knocked my car—and me—up onto the sidewalk just inches from a telephone pole.

That brought me to my senses, thankful I wasn't hurt.

It really is a good thing to take our problems to an all-wise Father. But under stress, I had disregarded the admonition that there is a time for everything.

Obviously, this was the time I should have been watching the traffic. Might I not have been as guilty of disregarding the lifesaver of temperance as was a drinking driver?

[1] Michael Young and Doug Williamson, in *Psychological Reports*, in *Reader's Digest*, December 1987, p. 34.

[2] J. C. Dousset, J. B. Gutierres, and N. Dousset, *The Lancet*, Dec. 13, 1986, p. 1393.

[3] William L. Weis, "Smoking and Unemployment," *Ministry*, Nov. 1987, p. 26.

[4] *Ibid.*, p. 27.

[5] Ralph Blodgett, *"Interview With Dr. C. Everett Koop, Surgeon General of the U.S.,"* *Vibrant Life*, November/December 1985, p. 18.

[6] J. Wayne McFarland, M.D., "How to Stop Smoking," special issue of *Vibrant Life*, pp. 16-19.

[7] U.S. Department of Health and Human Services, *For Good, a Guide to Living as a Nonsmoker*, p. 6.

[8] Mervyn G. Hardinge, *A Philosophy of Health*, p. 114.

[9] *Ibid.*

[10] *Ibid.*, p. 110.

[11] S. Gill and Associates, "Stroke and Alcohol Consumption," *The New England Journal of Medicine*, Oct. 16, 1986, p. 104.

[12] Interview with Greg Goodchild, director of the Clearview Alcohol and Drug Dependency Program of the Loma Linda Community Hospital, Loma Linda, California.

[13] Patricia Mutch, Ph.D., R.D., "Chemical Dependency: Impact on Youth," *Adventist Review*, Nov. 19, 1987, p. 10.

Lifesaver 4

REST

"What did you do today that was fun?" I asked the children as they came in from school.

"Oh, I wrote in my journal," 8-year-old Kristy answered. Her lips curved into a happy smile. "I wrote about our trip to Catalina—the boat, the waves, and all the fun we had." The older girls agreed they had enjoyed being with friends, and recess was nice, but they didn't exhibit the total joy of living that Kristy did.

Are you always in a hurry? Do you dash from one task to another, never taking time to enjoy what you're doing? I didn't realize how much of a clock-watcher I'd become until we were packing to come home after five years at a college in the Orient. As I dashed up to the administration building to turn in my final grades the dean of men came out of the dorm.

"Good morning, Mrs. Jones," he called.

"Hi! How are you?" I returned as I sped on my way.

"You're always in such a hurry," he commented. "In these five years I've never seen you walk. You always run."

"Come ye yourselves apart . . . and rest a while" (Mark 6:31).

"Oh, am I really that bad?" I wondered. I decided to check up on myself, fearing he might be right. He was right. I tended to hurry from one self-imposed task to another, to rush from one tiring day to the next.

I needed to do as Kristy—take time to enjoy life every step of the way.

I needed to remember to take time to live, time to think, time to smile, and time to play—time for just plain fun.

I should have slowed down years ago. But the strange thing is that I didn't realize what I was missing, rushing around as fast as I did, nor how much blood pressure and stress I was adding to the normal wear and tear of living.

How do you spend your leisure time? Bore-

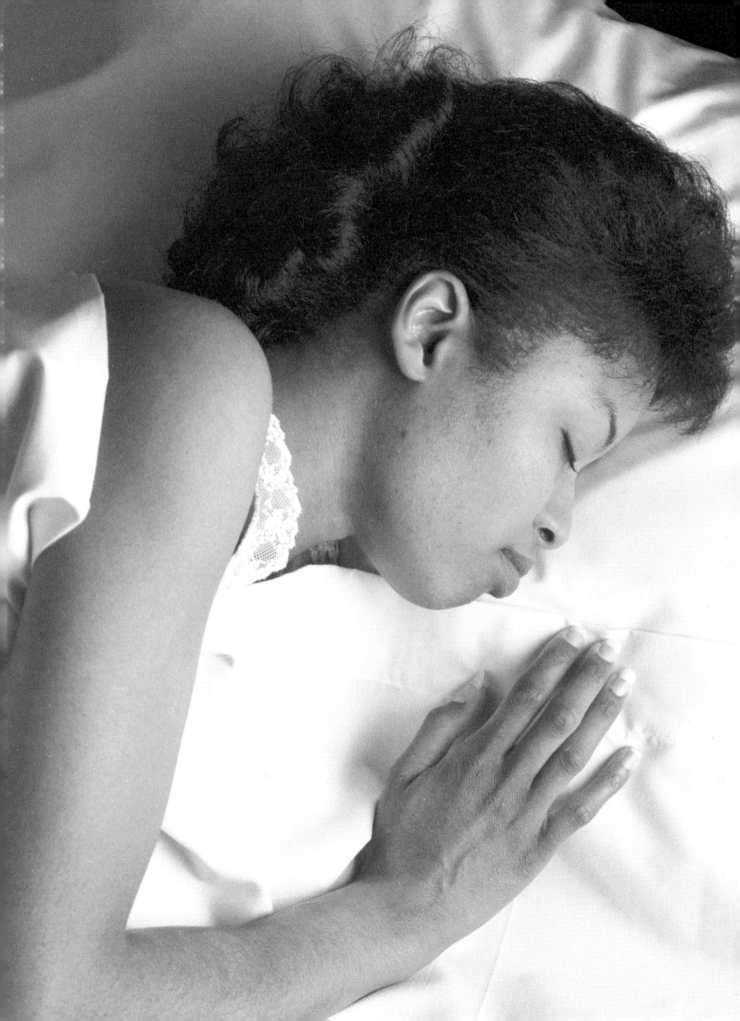

dom can produce stress, especially if you feel guilty for not accomplishing something important every minute. But if this is your thinking, maybe you, like I, need to revise your priorities.

Do you have a fun time with the children every evening before bedtime? And how about a family night once a week? Or a family weekend once a month? And a happy vacation every year?

These relaxed, fun times with your family may bring you greater dividends than you can imagine now. It is at such times that our social and spiritual values "rub off" onto the children, and husbands and wives fasten stronger ties to one another. Memories of these times together will strengthen and guide your children when they become teenagers and have to make some pretty important decisions—decisions that will determine their happiness and health throughout life.

Take rest; a field that has rested gives a bountiful crop."

Ovid

You don't always have to go to your bed and lie down in order to rest. A good spot on the carpet will do. Begin at your head and work your way down toward your toes.

Forcefully close your eyes, then relax those muscles. Do this several times. Then tighten the muscles in your neck and shoulders and relax them several times. Next, remember the little finger-play you used to do in kindergarten, holding your hands out in front: "Open, close them, open, close them, give a little clap. Open, close them, open, close them, put them in your lap." Just remember to make a tight fist when you close your hands.

First, proceed to tighten, then relax, the muscles of your arms, your abdomen, your legs, and your feet, doing each several times. Then take about 10 minutes or more just to lie there and enjoy that relaxed feeling.

How do you spend your evenings? And weekends? Do you grow tense watching frightening news reports of starving children, hostile engagements, calamities, or exciting ball games? Or do you take time to splice in an hour or two on your delightful hobby?

Remember, it's the activity that you thoroughly enjoy that is restful and may save your life.

Maybe you enjoy working on old cars, making one over into a shining exhibit of your skill and creative ability. Or how about painting? You don't to have to wait until you've retired, as Grandma Moses or Winston Churchill did. If you enjoy a musical instrument, take a little time out; let those tensions just run right out your fingers.

You would do well to have a hobby that gets you out with people. And you need one that you can enjoy alone on a rainy day when you want to stay home. You need one for summer when the sun shines and the flowers bloom and the birds sing. You need another for those cold winter days when you want to stay in your warm house.

Sewing, needlepoint, embroidery, knitting, crocheting, like painting, meet well your need for something restful and beautiful in your life.

No, these creative hobbies are not just for women. Dr. George Bowers, for 17 years president of Walla Walla College, once took a train trip to an important meeting in Washington, D.C. During the trip his seatmate, trying to be friendly, pulled a pack of cigarettes out of his pocket and offered him one.

"No, thank you. I don't smoke," President Bowers said.

The traveler puffed away on his for a while. Then he opened his briefcase and pulled out a deck of cards. "How about a game?" he suggested.

President Bowers shook his head with a smile. "No, thank you. I don't play cards," he replied.

The fellow seemed a little surprised and sat silent for a while. Then he got another idea. Pulling a flask from his hip pocket, he turned again to President Bowers and said, "Have a drink?"

"No, thank you. I don't drink."

"Then what do you do?" he exploded. "Knit?"

"Yes, as a matter of fact, I do," President Bowers surprised him.

President Bowers knit a number of elegant dresses for his wife, and many sweaters, which he gave away.

I treasure a woven yarn afghan that President Bowers made for me when he was in the hospital recovering from a heart attack. He seemed to enjoy this as much as the numerous items he made in his woodworking shop.

And then you must hear about the "mitten man" who lives near us.

When he moved south from Alaska, he continued this finger-warming project. To date, he has knit and given away to grateful friends over a thousand pairs of mittens.

Amateur radio can become a magical hobby, bringing you in contact with hams from all around the world. This can also help to meet your spiritual need. Six mornings a week my husband and I are up before six o'clock to join in the West Coast Bible Study Net. There we, with up to 50 other ham operators, join in a study that sets the tone of our day.

Another recreational hobby, fast growing among young and middle-aged persons, is that of RVing. Maybe you think that trailering or going by motor home or camper or tent is just for the old folks. But you'll quickly change your mind if you visit a state or national park between May and September. Parents and children are down there along the rivers and up there around the mountain lakes, fishing, hiking, or sitting on logs, just resting. Or they're out there in their sailboats, or skiing behind motorboats.

Your choice of a hobby can be a real lifesaver for you before the stresses you face can precipitate a heart attack or other emergency.

Most of us would do well to follow the example of the woman who was celebrating her one hundredth birthday. When someone asked her the reason for her long life, she replied, "When ah works, ah works hard; and when ah sits, ah sits loose-like."

Most of us need to learn to sit sort of "loose-like."

Dr. Charles Thomas, of the Banning Prevention Health Care and Educational Center, insists that you rest half an hour if you have a hydrotherapy treatment at his center. He says that during this half hour the number of your white cells in your blood increase dramatically.[1] This means that with all these germ fighters active your resistance to disease is greater. Next time you have a cold, try resting more. You may get well sooner.

When you are overly tired, you can't think straight. The wastes build up not only in your muscles but in your brain as well. Rest or a change of activity can help you to become more alert and refreshed.

To get the most from your sleep, you need to plan ahead and leave your work and problems at your workplace. The degree of rest you get from your sleep may depend on how much you can lay your burdens down and hand your cares over to the Life-giver.

Adequate sleep can help you to feel refreshed, with your mind keen, sharp, alert, and able to make wise decisions.

Getting plenty of sound sleep is a good way to program your 10 billion brain cells, more complicated than a modern computer, to flash the correct answer to your problems.

Rest and success are fellows."

W. G. Benham

How many hours of sleep did you get last night? Did you stay up watching the late show? Did you stay out at a party later than you'd planned? Did you pace the floor worrying over past mistakes? Or did you turn in at your regular early hour?

Dr. W. Proctor Harvey, of Georgetown University, classifies people into A, B, C, and D types. According to his grouping, if you are type A, you are alert and active in the morning and slow and inactive in the evening. Type B persons are more awake and active at night. Type C are good both times, and Type D, neither time.

He says, "We should pay attention to which type we are and, if possible, do our most important thinking and work during the time that we are alert, rather than at the time when we are sleepy and not really 'with it.' "[2]

Sleep is important because it builds up your body in so many ways. It rebuilds the cells of your muscles (including your heart muscle), your kidneys, bone marrow, stomach, and brain.

If you sprain an ankle, cut yourself, or break a bone, it will heal faster when you get extra sleep.

That's why it has been called the great restorer. Sleep prepares you for greater speed, accuracy, and efficiency both physically and mentally. It sweeps away fatigue and is one of nature's most effective brain fresheners. While you sleep, your blood and lymph systems continue to carry off the wastes to your skin, your kidneys, and your lungs, where they are eliminated. They also deposit in your brain a fresh supply of glucose and oxygen, which the cells must have for your brain to work well.

Shakespeare aptly referred to the "sleep that knits up the ravell'd sleave of care."

You experience two kinds of sleep: non-rapid eye movement (NREM) and rapid eye movement (REM). As you drop off to sleep you may feel a floating sensation or find your thoughts idly drifting.

Then within one to seven minutes you slip into a deeper sleep. You don't dream during these NREM stages of sleep. This is when

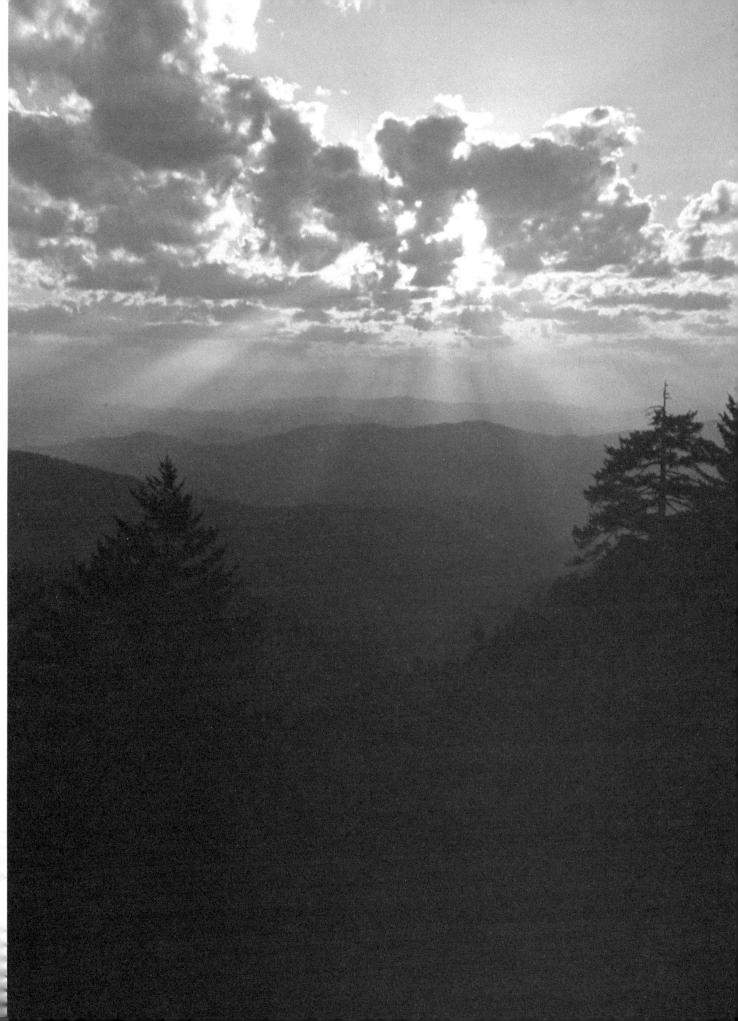

your muscles rejuvenate and your brain cells rest.

But as you move into the important rapid eye movement (REM) stage your brain becomes much more active. It sorts, analyzes, and files new information. This activity improves your learning ability and your memory, and helps you to make emotional and psychological adjustments. Here you solve problems and gain better perspective of difficult situations.[3] This REM stage of your sleep recurs approximately every 70 to 90 minutes after you go to sleep.[4] So you have four or five of these active brain periods each night. But it is interesting to note that toward morning the NREM stages shorten and REM sleep lengthens.

If you sleep only six hours your body may feel rested, but your brain needs those longer periods of REM sleep.[5] You should not take sleeping pills without your doctor's prescription, and then only when necessary. The use of barbiturates may keep you from dreaming, which is a most impartant part of normal sleep. Then you don't feel rested and will become more and more dependent upon medication.[6]

Most adults find they think more clearly and accomplish more when they have about eight hours of sleep. But you may require nine or ten for your best work.

When you are tempted to stay up and watch the late show, remember you can't replace your brain as you can a car battery, but you can go to sleep and recharge it. Some researchers believe that sleep even reinforces your character structure and that dreaming is necessary for you to maintain good mental health. A respected Bible teacher often coun-

seled his students: "Never make a major decision late at night. Wait until the next morning, when you are rested and your mind is clear."

Although you may not realize it, you dream about every 90 minutes while you sleep. Dreams seem to be an important factor in rapid learning and developing a good memory.

How much sleep do you need? You may feel you don't need as much as the average person, but your spouse probably could tell you that your disposition is the sweetest and you're more agreeable to live with when you regularly have from seven to nine hours of sleep. A sleepy person simply is not at his best, and the sleepier he is, the less effective will be his relationships and his productivity.

Sherry and Ted found out the hard way that caring for their bodies is important. As newlyweds, they thrilled at the thought of working together in an overseas mission. Both, having been trained for the work in which they were to engage, could scarcely wait to start packing. But her physical examination revealed that Sherry was unfit for the assignment. She was totally unsuited physically and emotionally for the job.

Heartsick, she confessed that throughout her college years she had carried a heavy load with far too little rest. This took its toll, and the price she paid was failure to realize her greatest ambition—serving in the mission field.

Michelle was more fortunate, though she learned through a hard experience.

Early in the school year she stayed a few minutes after class to talk with me. She seemed so nervous and fidgety that I invited her into my office and asked if I could help her.

Right away she burst out in fear, "I'm afraid they're going to send me home."

"Why would they send you home?" I wondered aloud.

"Oh, I'm failing my courses. And I know they're going to send me home." She turned her face so I wouldn't see the tears slipping down her cheeks.

"Are you studying your lessons?"

"Yes."

"How much?" I asked.

"Oh, I study all the time. I just study all the time."

"Do you eat breakfast?"

"No. I don't have time to. I study my math during the breakfast hour."

"How much sleep do you get?"

"Not much. I have too much to do," Michelle said.

"Are you taking a gym class?"

"No. I need that time to study."

"Have you taken a walk, a run, or a bicycle ride today?"

She looked at me with eyes that seemed to say "How foolish can you be?"

We talked about the value of sunshine, fresh air, exercise, time for personal devotions, plenty of good nourishment, water, and rest. I explained to her that the more she studied, the more her brain needed rest and a change of activity. The more her muscles sat idle, the more they cried out for action. The more she worked and used up her blood sugar, the more she needed nourishment.

Several studies show that physical exercise in the form of a gym class, swimming, or other aerobic exercise is not a waste of time. It is an advantage because it makes your brain more alert.

Then I urged her to go to her room, sit down, and make out a schedule for every day of the week, beginning with a personal devotional time every morning. Then plan for at least two good meals and no in-between-meal snacks, to include time for outdoor recreation, and a quiet study time for each lesson.

"Come back next week and let me know how it goes," I told her.

"I'll try. And thanks," she said as she hurried to her next assignment.

When I met Michelle in the hall a few days later, I didn't need to ask any questions. She beamed as she volunteered, "Oh, I'm doing a lot better. I passed two quizzes already, and I think they're going to let me stay." They did, and she did!

Michelle's brain and body worked together to prepare for her a successful career.

You too will find that your brain works best in a strong body.

When you feel well, and thus feel good about yourself, you can accomplish much more in the same length of time and without getting so tired.

Research analysts tell us that if you can't go to sleep until very late some night, you shouldn't lie there and pity yourself and make excuses when it's time to get up the next morning. Get up at your regular time. You'll be more likely to get to sleep right on time the next night.

If you take long flights, crossing several time zones, you may have a much easier time adjusting your sleep pattern to the new schedule if you make your flight in the daytime.

(But alas, most of the overseas flights seem to be at night.)

You may be better able to plan your schedule after arrival if you realize that you will be likely to adapt after your westward flight more readily than after your eastward trip.

The more you participate in local life, the more quickly you will likely adapt to local time. Apparently social factors and scheduling greatly affect your body rhythm adaptation.[7] If you happen to work a night shift and are off one or two nights, you may find that your brain and body function better if you adhere as far as feasible to your regular sleep schedule. Even on a daytime schedule we seem to work best and feel better when we maintain regularity in our daily program of rest, activity, and eating.

If you have a hard time going to sleep, there are a number of things to try before resorting to sleeping pills and risking the danger of developing drug dependency.

1. Start for bed at a regular time each night.

2. Take a warm shower.

3. Darken the room and adjust the temperature.

4. Open a window for fresh air.

5. Turn off all sounds, unless you are one who has to have the hum of an electric fan, the ticking of a clock, or the sound of traffic.

6. Read something calming, preferably your Bible or other spiritually encouraging book.

7. Lay your burdens down. Sometimes we remember to give our financial gifts to God but forget to give Him our burdens as well.

Dr. O. A. Battista, a research chemist, clears his brain for sleep. "My personal routine," he says, "is to imagine a wastebasket beside the bed, and as each cluttering thought comes to mind I mentally discard it by tossing it into the wastebasket. As soon as the basket is full and my mind is empty, I'm off to slumberland."

When I have an occasional problem of getting to sleep, I like to start with "A" and quote a Bible promise that begins with each letter of the alphabet until I get to "Z"—or "ZZZ-Z-Z-Z," whichever comes first.

Grab a hold on the lifesaver SLEEP and hang on there.

---

[1] Interview with Charles S. Thomas, D.P.H., Nov. 23, 1987.
[2] W. Proctor Harvey, M.D., "Sleep—Absence Makes the Heart Grow Fonder," *Medical Times*, June 1979, p. 17.
[3] Jean Hayter, R.N., Ed.D., "The Rhythm of Sleep," *American Journal of Nursing*, March 1980, p. 458.
[4] Kristine Adam, B.Sc., "A Time for Rest and a Time for Play," *Nursing Mirror*, Mar. 6, 1980, p. 17.
[5] Hayter.
[6] *Medical Times*, vol. 107, No. 6, p. 32.
[7] Elliot D. Weitzman, M.D., and Charles P. Pollak, M.D., "Disorders of the Circadian Sleep-Wake Cycle," *Medical Times*, June 1979, p. 85.

EXERCISE

"John came home feeling tense, anxious, and irritable. He was a manager for a large business firm, and had spent all day, trying unsuccesfully to mend sharp differences between two of his key department heads. After fighting traffic for 45 minutes on the way home, he felt he needed to clear his mind.

"Slipping on his well-worn jogging shoes, John went out for a 30-minute jog through the dirt trails behind his house. By the time he returned home, he felt completely different. His mind felt relaxed, his mood was elevated, and all his built-up tension was erased. After stretching and showering, John enjoyed the evening with his family.

"Donna felt depressed. She had just received a low C on her first biochemistry test, and as a freshman medical student, she was extremely worried about her chances of staying in the program. Pulling on her jacket, she went out for a 40-minute brisk walk on the hilly roads near her school. By the time

Donna returned to her dorm room, her spirits were lifted, her depression was gone, and she sat down at her desk with renewed determination to keep pressing on with her studies." [1]

Can exercise really do this much for mental anxiety and depression? As you read this chapter you may be surprised to learn the wonderful benefits of exercise.

Richard Kegley, twice acclaimed world champion runner for his age group, declares there are many benefits to be gained from a regular exercise program.

For him it meant dropping to his ideal weight, which gave him increased strength and endurance. He says, "The allergies, asthma, and medicines are gone. My blood pressure is 120/70. My doctor says that's excellent. Running has built up my resistance, too. Another thing—today I can read material that I have read many times, but see things in it that I never saw there before." [2]

Are you interested in exercise for the pur-

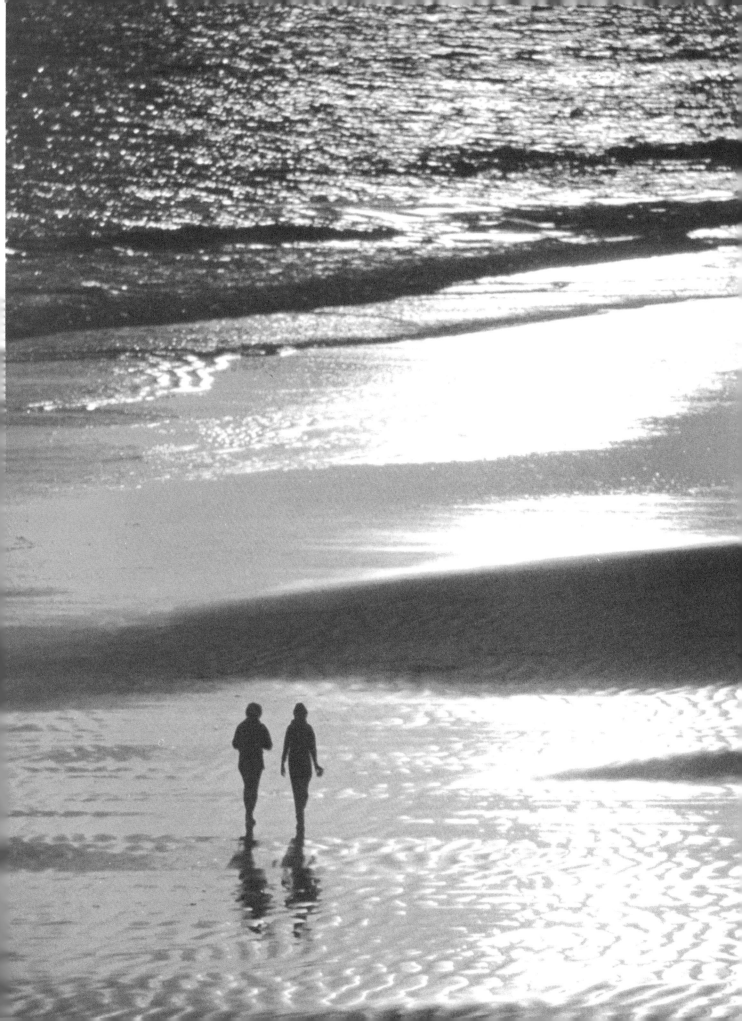

pose of losing weight? If you are, you will be happy to know that exercise taken in the morning results in greater weight loss than the same amount taken at night.[3] Another advantage of scheduling your exercise for the morning is that you are more likely to get it done. If you plan it for the evening, you have all day long to let something else slip in to keep you from doing it.

Dr. Lee S. Berk, assistant research professor of pathology, Loma Linda University, Loma Linda, California, found that "in runners and other routine exercisers, an endocrine hormone called beta-endorphin becomes elevated differently than in sedentary people. A natural opiate (pain-killing) substance, beta-endorphin not only kills pain and makes you feel good but also helps reduce your blood pressure, heart rate, and respiration."[4,5,6]

If you or someone in your family is a student, encourage him to register for a class in swimming. This is an excellent aerobic exercise, and a study of those who engage in it reports they have less tension, depression, anger, and confusion, and more vigor, than those who were not swimmers.[7]

Other reports indicate, as did the experience of Dick Kegley, the runner, that memory and intellectual functions are improved by a walk/jog program.[8] Several researchers have discovered that during exercise we have an increase in alpha waves. These are the brain waves that are associated with a relaxed, meditation-like state. They feel this helps to explain how exercise reduces anxiety and depression.[9]

So next time you feel "blue," depressed, or

under stress, you may find relief by a vigorous walk in the fresh air.

Physiologists have found also that when you exercise, your bone marrow makes red cells at a faster rate. This is significant, because red blood cells carry fresh oxygen to your brain and all parts of your body.

Another good thing that exercise does is to speed up the flow of lymph, removing the waste products that otherwise would make you feel sluggish.

If you want to know if your brain is flabby, feel your legs."
Bruce Barton

Not only running or jogging, but other simple exercises can help you feel better. If you sit at your work, you may find that alternate shrugging and relaxing of your shoulders several times is an easy way to relieve tension, pain, and headaches. Getting up and walking around at least once every hour is important to prevent blood clots.

Next time you're uptight, try taking a brisk walk. Instead of becoming more tired and tense, you will find yourself unwinding. Nathan Pritikin explained to his patients that inactive muscles build up strong electrical charges that keep one awake, but with exercise "you can discharge those voltages, and muscles relax. Dissipating those electrical charges in the muscles is precisely what tranquilizers do." Just think how much better a brisk walk is for you than are tranquilizers with all their side effects.

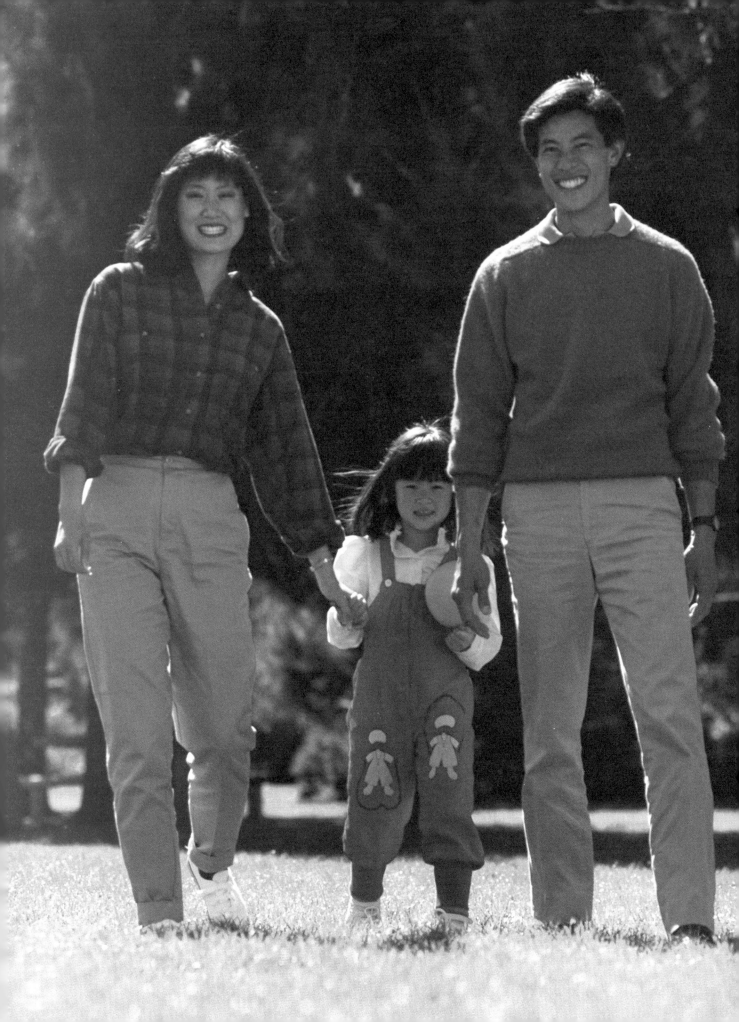

We need to balance our emotions with motion. How can we do that?

Suppose you become angry or upset at your spouse or someone else. Instead of fighting and saying harsh words that you will later regret, you can go out and play a game of tennis together to build up those happiness hormones. The exercise will use up the excess electrical charges your anger has produced, calm your emotions, and as a result, strengthen your relationship.

One Christian writer even suggests that if you are angry, you might get more good out of chopping a load of wood than by sitting through a prayer meeting.

Are you wondering how much exercise is enough? For different people the answer will be different, because it depends on just what you want from your exercise. If you want to be a champion runner, then you're going to have to do a lot of running. You would need to get your doctor's advice and carefully watch your progress, weighing it, your health, and your goals.

However, to get the most good out of your exercise, the set of your mood needs to be right.

If you are a sedentary person, you probably can extend your life several years by regular aerobic exercise, such as brisk walking, running, swimming, or cycling.

But if you consider yourself neither sedentary nor active, just somewhere in between, there is good news for you, too. Recent research at the University of Minnesota School of Public Health "found that men at high risk for heart disease who engage in moderate exercise can reduce their risk of dying from a heart attack by as much as one third over a seven-year period." They did this simply by moderate exercise such as rapid walking, gardening, yard work, home repairs, and home exercise for about an hour a day.[10]

> Scientists now readily agree that there is a much closer relationship between your mind and your body than most of us realize. When either is affected, the other is also.

It is interesting to know that the same amount of exercise that helps your heart also helps your brain.

Dr. Mervyn G. Hardinge, of the Loma Linda School of Health, Loma Linda, California, reports on a study he did. Notice the close relationship between the mental attitudes of these participants and their physiological reactions.

The wise for cure on exercise depend."
Dryden

"We divided the group so that when half of them were exercising, the other half were resting. The exercise consisted of two kinds. During the exercise period, one half worked on the treadmill and the other half did 'fun' exercises—anything they liked to do just so it required vigorous activity. For the second exercise period, those who had been on the treadmill now played tennis or did some other enjoyable exercise while those who had done 'fun' exercises now worked on the treadmill."

When the experiment was finished, every student reported which exercise he enjoyed and which he didn't. Students who enjoyed the exercise lowered their blood cholesterol levels. Those who did not enjoy it maintained their control levels.

Some enjoyed the games but not the treadmill; others enjoyed the treadmill but not the games. Some enjoyed both. Those who enjoyed both lowered their cholesterol levels the most.

"The conclusion is obvious. You must enjoy your leisure time to derive the most benefit. Your exercise must be vigorous, but not one which causes tension or excessive drive." [11]

Whether you choose to run, jog, walk, bike, swim, or just work in your garden, you will find enjoyable activity an excellent Lifesaver.

---

[1] David Nieman, D.H.Sc., M.P.H., *The Sports Medicine Fitness Course* (Palo Alto, Calif.: Bull Pub. Co., 1986), p. 250.

[2] Personal interviews with Richard Kegley, from 1985 through 1987.

[3] Nieman, p. 322.

[4] Nieman, p. 254.

[5] Interview with Lee S. Berk, D.H.Sc., M.P.H., F.A.C.S.M., Loma Linda University, Loma Linda, California, Dec. 11, 1987.

[6] Mike Schwartz, in Riverside (California) *Press Enterprise*, Nov. 9, 1987, Section C.

[7] Nieman, p. 253.

[8] *Ibid.*

[9] *Ibid.*, p. 255.

[10] "How Much Exercise Is Enough?" *University of California Wellness Letter*, January 1988, p. 1.

[11] Mervyn G. Hardinge, *A Philosophy of Health* (Loma Linda, Calif.: Loma Linda University, 1980), p. 35. Used by permission.

Lifesaver 6

A GOOD DIET

As I totaled up the score and placed the grade at the top of Roger's health-science test I looked again at the name. Surely it couldn't be Roger's paper! He always earned a good grade. Again I added the figures and checked the name. It really was Roger's paper, and he had earned only a D. I decided that he must have been sick.

When Roger came to class the next morning I whispered as I handed his paper to him, "What happened to you?"

I expected his eyes to drop and a disappointed look to cross his face as he caught sight of the grade. But instead he grinned and said, "It worked."

"What worked? What were you trying to do?"

"Well, you see," he explained, "I wondered if what you said was true, and I found out. Usually I eat a good breakfast, but yesterday I decided to see for myself if skipping breakfast really would make any difference in my ability to remember what I had studied. From now on I eat breakfast!"

A good diet begins with a good breakfast. For a breakfast that will keep you feeling alert and energetic all morning, try one that includes a citrus fruit or juice, one other fruit, whole-grain cereal or bread, low-fat milk or yogurt, peanut butter or a high-protein food such as a meat analog.

Several years ago when I was lecturing about breakfasts to a college health class, the son of a prominent doctor spoke up: "We eat dinner at breakfast time. We wouldn't want to go back to the old way for anything."

This was a new idea to me, but as I questioned him further I found they had a sound nutritional plan. So I kept my ears open to learn how others got adequate protein at breakfast. I learned of a Bible teacher, a salesman, a nutritionist, a nurse, and their families who also regularly had "dinner" at breakfast time.

47

My husband and I concluded that this must be worth testing, so we decided to give it a try for a month. And guess what! At the end of four weeks we too liked it. We found that at breakfast time our stomachs felt more in the mood to take more food than at noon or evening. We also discovered that we ended up having a better dinner than when we ate later in the day.

I could plan our meal the evening before, place items to be baked in the oven when I got up in the morning, and have a hot dinner ready by breakfast time.

We find that on this program we have more energy throughout the morning and accomplish our work more easily. We are more cheerful and are better able to cope with whatever problems arise during the day. If you wonder how you could eat that much food so early in the day, try eating little or nothing in the evening. Then the next morning take a good walk, a run, or a jog before breakfast.

As I continued to learn about the importance of breakfast I discovered that schoolchildren who eat a really good breakfast stay more alert and concentrate better on their schoolwork than children who eat a skimpy breakfast. I wish we had known this when our children were young.

A study of the efficiency of factory workers shows that breakfast eaters produced more and suffered fewer accidents during the hour just before lunch than did their counterparts who ate poor breakfasts.[1]

What accounts for these changes in behavior, attitude, and physical achievement?

The accompanying chart contrasts the blood sugar levels of those who eat a good breakfast with the blood sugar levels of those who eat a poor breakfast.

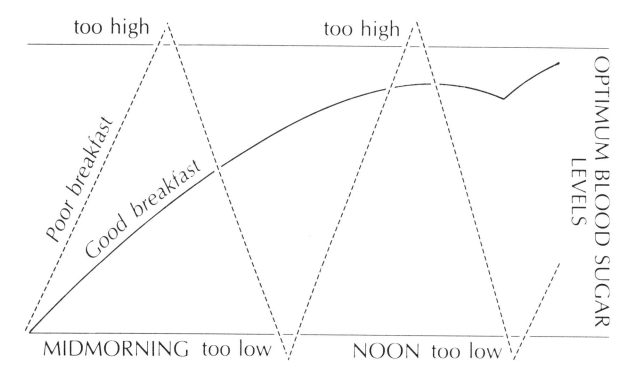

When you have a breakfast composed chiefly of refined carbohydrates (like a sweet bun and a sweetened cup of coffee, or a piece of white bread with jam and a glass of orange juice), your blood sugar increases very rapidly. In fact, it goes up so fast that the pancreas must send out an emergency supply of insulin. The insulin acts so promptly to take care of the extra amount of sugar that your blood sugar level drops dramatically.

By midmorning you feel so hungry that you take another cup of coffee with sugar, and a couple of cookies. Again your blood sugar shoots up, and is counteracted with another spurt of insulin. By lunchtime you are weak, tired, and accident-prone. You may even have a headache. Because you feel so ill, you grab a doughnut and another cup of coffee (with sugar for a quick lift), and light a cigarette. Thus you set the stage for a repeat performance during the afternoon.

And sure enough, by midafternoon you have to rush out for another shot of sugar and caffeine, probably a Coke. By 5:00, when you head home for a heavy dinner, you are the picture of fatigue and feel like an old grouch. Do you recognize yourself in this habit pattern?

There are a number of dangers to this type of diet that thousands, perhaps millions, of Americans follow.

Since the brain depends entirely on glucose for its activity, anything that drops the sugar content of the blood below normal levels affects the operation of your brain cells. No wonder so many people have problems!

Such a diet also overworks the pancreas and may initiate the onset of diabetes.

If you eat a heavy meal at night just before going to bed, you don't burn up your dinner calories. They produce fat, some of which becomes embedded in the blood vessel walls—especially in the heart and brain—weakening them and laying the groundwork for heart attack or stroke.

Caring for a big meal overworks your tired digestive system and results in restless sleep. It also calls the blood from your head to your stomach, and again you cannot think as clearly and reason as well as you should. Perhaps this is one reason many psychologists urge people not to make major decisions in the evening.

Now back to the chart. Take a look at the line representing the blood-sugar level when you have a good breakfast with adequate protein. The fruit supplies enough energy to get you off to a good start. The unrefined cereals, as they are absorbed and metabolized, continue to keep the blood sugar up to a good level. Then, considerably later, the proteins are broken down and continue to supply your needs.

Benefits of a High Protein Breakfast

1. Greater maximum work before lunch.
2. Better sustained mental alertness.
3. Less muscular fatigue.
4. Greater endurance.
5. Less accident-prone output.
6. Less oxygen required to produce given amount of work.
7. Less neuromuscular tremor.
8. Less nervous irritability.

Sample Breakfasts

Breakfast No. 1

Soy or whole-wheat waffles with peanut butter and applesauce
Half a grapefruit
A glass of nonfat milk
One serving of scrambled Egg Beaters, or other egg substitute

Breakfast No. 2

Hash-brown potatoes (browned with Pam or very little oil)
Scrambled tofu*
Whole-wheat toast
Margarine (optional)
Half glass of orange juice
Half glass of nonfat milk
Apple

Breakfast No. 3

Granola (including grains, nuts, and fruit)*
Fruit yogurt
One cup nonfat milk
Whole-wheat toast
Soft margarine (optional)
An orange

_____

*See appendix for recipe.

And now that you have breakfast behind you, what about the rest of the day? What more should you have to meet the rest of your needs?

One easy way is to take a glance at this chart and choose at least:

(Group 1)

Two servings of nonfat milk, milk products, or milk substitutes. This group supplies liberal amounts of calcium, phosphorus, protein, and riboflavin.

(Group 2)

Two servings of protein foods such as beans, lentils, tofu, or low-fat cottage cheese, nuts, peanut butter, or meat analogs. (More and more supermarkets now carry these meat substitutes.) A good variety supplies all the protein you need for building tissue and antibodies.

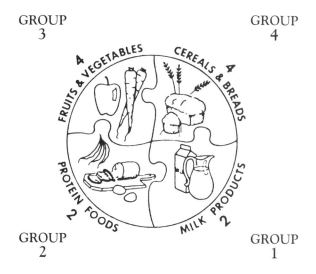

(Group 3)

Four servings of fruits and vegetables. Include one citrus fruit or other food rich in vitamin C; also one leafy green or dark-yellow vegetable or yellow fruit as a source of vitamin A. (It is better to eat your fruit and vegetables at different meals.) These are called protective foods because of their generous vitamin, mineral, and fiber content.

(Group 4)

Four servings of grain products, such as oatmeal, brown rice, whole-wheat bread, and unrefined breakfast cereals.

These provide B vitamins, iron, phosphorus, and proteins.

Did you know that you can eat the recommended number of servings from each of the four food groups and still not have an optimal diet?

So you still need to use good judgment and choose the less refined foods and few sweets. For instance, in group 4 (cereals) you could choose whole-grain bread, white bread, or sugared doughnuts. In group 1 (milk), you might have milk, sweet fruit-flavored yogurt, or canned chocolate pudding. And group 2 (proteins), cooked soybeans, tofu, or soy chocolate fudge. Group 3 (fruits and vegetables) could include corn on the cob, canned creamed corn, or caramel popcorn.

A great **deal of poor health in this country may be attributed to heavy meals and light work."**

We give caution against the frequent use of ripened yellow cheese and high-fat milk, for recent findings reveal a positive relationship of these items with cancer.[2]

Probably you have noticed that not only *what* you eat, but *when* you eat affects your health.

One of the easiest ways to cut down on sweets is to leave off between-meal snacks.

Dr. Thayer, a California State University psychologist, did a study comparing the energy received from a candy bar and that from a 10-minute walk. He reports "walking was associated with higher self-rated energy and lower tension significantly more than was snacking. The sugar snack . . . was associated with tense energy and then tense tiredness for a majority of the participants."

After eating the candy bar, subjects said they felt more tired and more tense than before the snack. The walk gave the participants much more energy and lessened their tension for up to two hours.[3] This suggests that if you have had adequate food, you may feel more refreshed by a 10-minute walk than by a between-meal snack. Why not try it? Sounds like a great lifesaver to me.

But why do you enjoy sweets so much? Maybe you simply loved sweets the first time you tasted them. Some nutritionists disagree. But most of us develop a taste for sweets early in life.

Actually, we are trained to like sweets, if we didn't from the first. Adults smile and smack their lips and comment on how good, yummy, and delicious they are when they give them to us as toddlers.

We then had our pleasure response to the sweet. Often sugar is made into the most attractive food on the table, so this adds to its appeal. The calorie content is high, and this gives us a lift and a satisfied feeling.

But you are smart enough to weigh the case against sugar before using it too freely.

As my husband and I waited for transportation in Los Angeles, a mother with a 5-

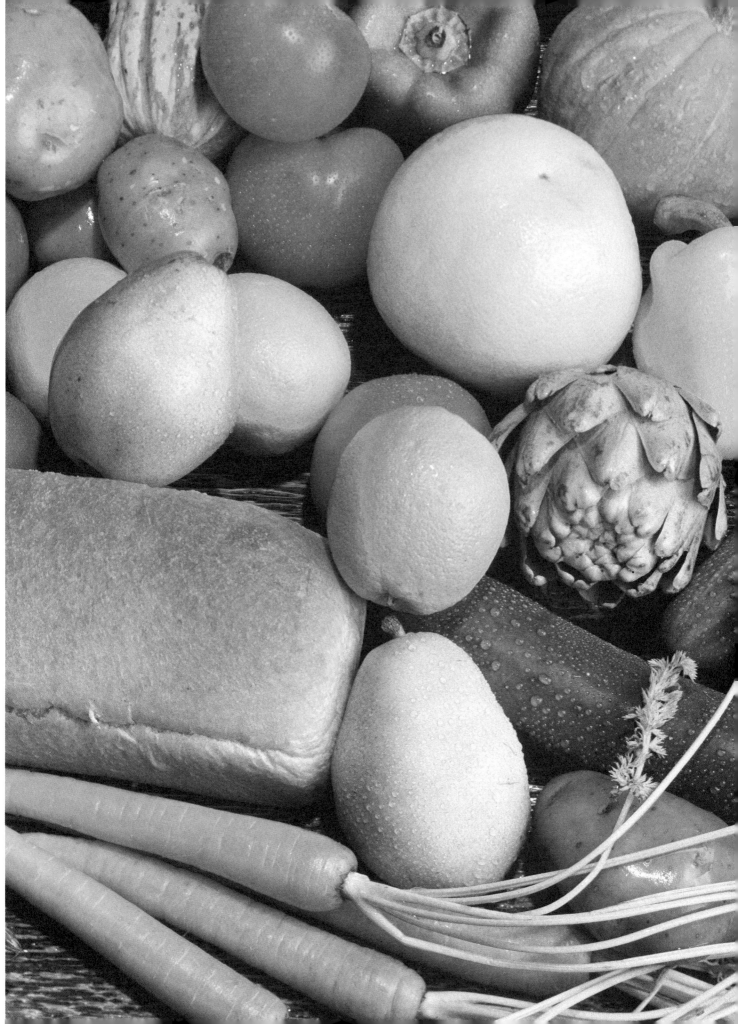

month-old baby sat down beside us. She put the little fellow in his infant seat and set it on the floor. He appeared very restless and tired. I wanted to change his position and give him a rest, but his mother didn't seem to think of that.

Shortly she reached into her satchel and pulled out a can of Coke, yanked the tab open, dropped a straw into it, sucked the straw full, then put her finger over the upper end and placed the other into the helpless baby's mouth, allowing the liquid to run down his throat. The infant frowned and wrinkled his tiny face while he tried to turn his head away, as if to say "Don't do that to me!" But the well-meaning but ignorant mother continued trying to make her baby accept the Coke.

Caffeinated beverages and chocolate confections can readily jeopardize the health of children. A bottle of warm milk, or even tap water, would have helped that poor baby, whereas the caffeine and temperature of the Coke could only keep him awake, making him more restless and uncomfortable.

And why do you want to cut down on sweets? Of course, one reason is the soaring dental bills that go along with increased cavities. Drs. Weiss and Trithart studied a group of 783 children 5 to 6 years of age in relation to between-meal eating habits and dental caries. They discovered that those children who ate nothing between meals had many fewer cavities than those who snacked. The accompanying chart shows the rewards of not eating between meals.[4]

Another reason you want to cut down on the sweets you give your children is that sugar greatly slows down the activity of your white blood cells—germ fighters. Thus a high level of sugar in the diet weakens resistance to colds and other diseases.

The human body, with proper care, will last a lifetime.

A young mother of three children said to me, "I never imagined that cutting down on sweets could make such a difference in my children. They're so calm! They get along better together and aren't nearly so fussy." She'd recently heard of the benefits of a low-sugar diet and had tested it on her family.

Did you know that for every grain of sugar you eat, you use vitamin B_1 (thiamine) to burn it up and release energy? Thiamine is sometimes called the happiness vitamin, for when we don't have enough of it, we become irritable. The more sweets we eat, the more thiamine we need, but most of the refined

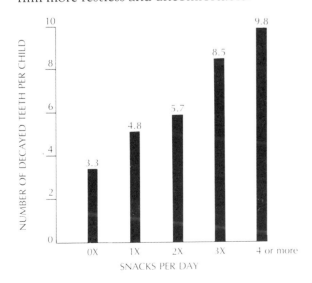

pastries we get have little or no thiamine. No wonder a diet high in refined carbohydrates affects the disposition. Too bad that the bride often thinks her culinary expertise in the area of pies, cakes, cookies, and candy will win her the admiration of her new husband! Unfortunately, these very things may sour his disposition and make the bride more irritable too.

We have already noted that blood sugar shoots up and down with a sweet breakfast and between-meal sweets. Think for a moment how you feel when your energy level is high. You get "itchy feet." You want to get going. You have a host of great ideas for things you want to do right away.

Now suppose your son, Jimmy, is at this point. A friend comes along with a suggestion that he skip school, smoke a cigarette, try a marijuana joint, or do any one of a dozen other things that normally would not tempt him. Unless he has learned strong moral reasoning, unless he has already made a decision *never* to do those certain things, he may have a problem. When his body is crying out for activity and excitement, he is less likely to stop and think through the situation. He is too eager for action. He has energy to burn. It is easy to tumble for the temptation without a second thought.

Or consider the other extreme—when his blood sugar reaches its lowest point. His vitamin B_1 is pretty low. His energy is low. He feels tired. He thinks slowly. He's hungry and doesn't care what happens. And so Jimmy has another susceptible moment. When the nutrition (glucose) in his brain is depleted, his brain cells don't function well. And remember, his brain cells are the only medium through which his conscience can communicate with him. When he feels low, he may easily be tempted to steal a candy bar or steal money to buy a doughnut or bottle of pop. Then when his blood sugar begins to climb, he feels so good that the guilt seems just to dissolve away.

Does this help you to understand that a perverted appetite can help you to lose your power to resist temptation? You can see why some people are termed "candy criminals."

The Inter-Society Commission for Heart Disease Resources recommends for your heart's sake that you progress to "a more vegetarian diet without excess calories" because this can lower your cholesterol.[5] And isn't it comforting to know, when you sit down and look at your food, that you don't have to wonder what disease it died of? Of course, you are aware that many sick chickens and animals are rushed to the market before they die.

Do you tire easily when you run, jog, walk, or work? If so, you will be interested to know how you can increase your endurance.[6]

David Nieman, D.H.Sc., exercise physiologist at Loma Linda University, says, "The latest studies have concentrated on the importance of carbohydrates in the diet. Vegetarian diets can easily provide for the high-carbohydrate intake that can double or triple endurance time."[6]

Benefits of a Vegetarian Diet

1. Has less cholesterol.
2. Has less total fat and less saturated fat.
3. Provides greater endurance.
4. Has fewer calories, so adds fewer excess pounds.

5. Is more economical.
6. Is less likely to cause cancer and other diet-related disease.
7. Provides increased vitamins, minerals, and fiber.

Dr. Scharffenberg also says your risk of heart attacks can be reduced by 90 percent, chiefly by not smoking and by using a vegetarian diet, which can also "reduce your risk of cancer, diabetes, osteoporosis, and a whole host of diseases."

And if you are concerned that on a vegetarian diet you might not get enough protein, you will be interested to learn that

1. "The quality of protein in brown rice ranks slightly higher than that of red muscle meat.

2. "Ten percent of the calories in your potato and 35 percent of those in your serving of broccoli come in the form of quality protein.

3. "Four to 6 percent of the calories in fruit is protein, and many of the foods you eat for iron, vitamins, or energy sneak you a little protein each time you eat them."

"Even more important, you will have greater endurance and feel much better. You will enjoy a much wider variety of the most appetizing foods and note an improvement in quality of life." [7]

To Save Your Heart

1. Cut down on sweets.
2. Use fewer fatty foods.
3. Maintain optimum weight.
4. Eat a low-salt, low-cholesterol diet.
5. Substitute soy proteins for meat.

David Snowden, Ph.D., an epidemiologist at the University of Minnesota, reported on a 21-year study of 25 Seventh-day Adventists. "In both males and females, the higher the egg consumption, the higher the rate of colon cancer. Prostate cancer in males appears to be tripled by the combined use of meat, milk, eggs, and cheese."

There is a great deal of discussion today about the relation of fiber to cancer of the colon, because adequate fiber roughage in the diet can cut in half the time food takes to travel from the mouth through your digestive system. Many researchers feel that the shorter the time the food stays in the colon, the less likelihood one has of cancer.

As fiber attaches to the cholesterol in the colon, it keeps the cholesterol from being absorbed into the blood and clogging up the blood vessels. [9]

Inasmuch as heart and blood-vessel disease is the number one killer in the United States, we all do well to learn all we can about preventing it in our families.

Dr. Scharffenberg says the following practice can greatly cut your risk of coronary heart disease:

Cut down on foods high in cholesterol, saturated fats, calories, sugar, and salt. Some of the foods high in cholesterol are eggs, beef steaks and roasts, hamburgers, meat loaves, whole milk, hot dogs, ham, and luncheon meats. [10]

"People have for some years been buying purified fiber to sprinkle onto their foods in the hope of improving their health. But the purified fiber they buy most often is wheat bran, the type with the least cholesterol-lowering effect. Fibers better at lowering blood cholesterol include pectin and gums —found in greater abundance in fruits, vegetables, and legumes, rather than grains.[11]

Now you will be happy to find out something else you can easily do to prevent building up cholesterol deposits in your blood vessels. Dr. James Blankenship, of the Department of Nutrition, Loma Linda University School of Nutrition, says recent research has found that "contributing factors of heart disease are reduced by the consumption of olive oil. The arteries of olive oil-fed animals have aged less than those fed other fats. The arteries are more pliable, more elastic, and therefore able to respond to the pressure.

"Factors that tend to reduce high blood pressure are increased by consumption of olive oil."[12] Sounds like something worth trying, doesn't it?

Now to make your selection of foods easiest Dr. John Scharffenberg offers a one-sentence university course in nutrition: Eat at proper times a variety of natural foods in quantities to maintain ideal weight.[13]

---

[1] Thomas R. Hood, M.D., M.P.H., Kansas State Board of Health, radiobroadcast 2629 on station KVOE.

[2] M. G. Lee, L. H. Moulton, C. Hill, and A. Kramer, "Consumption of Dairy Products and Alcohol in Breast Cancer," *Journal of the National Cancer Institute*, September 1986, p. 633.

[3] In *The Informer*, Pacific Press Publishing Association newsletter, Nov. 10, 1987, p. 4; reprinted from the *Journal of Personality and Social Psychology* 52, No. 1 (1987).

[4] Robert L. Weiss, D.D.S., M.P.H., F.A.P.H.A., and Albert H. Trithart, D.D.S., M.P.H., F.A.P.H.A., "Between-Meal Eating Habits and Dental Caries Experience in Preschool Children," *American Journal of Public Health*, August 1960, p. 1097.

[5] J. A. Scharffenberg, M.D., *Diet and Heart Disease*, 1987, p. 7, quoted from: *Report of Inter-Society Commission for Heart Disease Resources. Circulation 70 (1984)*: 157A-205A.

[6] Robert Kowalski, M.S., Patricia K. Johnston, M.S., R.D., Kenneth I. Burke, Ph.D., and Harley Stanton, M.P.H., "Congress Investigates Vegetarian Nutrition, *Nutrition Today*, July/August 1987.

[7] Scharffenberg, p. 23.

[8] David Snowden, Ph.D., "Vegetarian Diets and Mortality," *Nutrition Today*, July/August 1987.

[9] Scharffenberg, p. 18.

[10] *Ibid.*, p. 2.

[11] Eleanor Noss Whitney and Eva May Nunnelley Hamilton, *Understanding Nutrition*, 4th ed. (New York: West Pub. Co., 1987), p. 104.

[12] Interview with James Blankenship, Ph.D., Department of Nutrition, Loma Linda University, Loma Linda, California, Dec. 18, 1987.

[13] Scharffenberg, p. 21.

Lifesaver 7

WATER

My guest looked at his watch, then asked, "May I have a drink of water, please?"

"Surely."

Then as I started for the refrigerator, he added, "Oh, tap water's just fine. Thanks."

Lisa, his wife, looked at her watch and said, "I think I'll take one too, please."

I looked at my kitchen clock. *Nothing unusual about 12:10*, I thought. *We'll be eating lunch in about half an hour.* And I gave them each a drink.

A half hour later, I set glasses on the table and poured water into them for lunch. Both Lisa and Hal spoke up and said that they didn't care for any.

I said, "OK," but poured some for the rest of us.

As we chatted and enjoyed our meal I noticed they both ate rather slowly, thoroughly chewing each bite.

I sat there drinking more water while waiting for them to finish the meal.

Lisa insisted on helping me clear the table and straighten up the kitchen, saying she was used to taking a little exercise after eating.

An hour or two later she was ready for another drink. *Well*, I thought, *you seem to live by the clock. Why do you drink at specific times? I drink when I'm thirsty.*

Lisa seemed to read my thoughts. "We find our digestion is better if we don't drink water with our meals, but we drink enough in between times so we don't miss it at the table."

As I thought about it, it didn't take me long to realize there is common sense in Lisa's and Bill's drinking habit. When you drink a lot of water with your meals, the liquid dilutes the saliva in your mouth, the gastric juice in your stomach, and the digestive juices in the upper part of your intestines.

Then when I left off the water at meals, I found I chewed my food much better, mixing it thoroughly with my saliva, which was

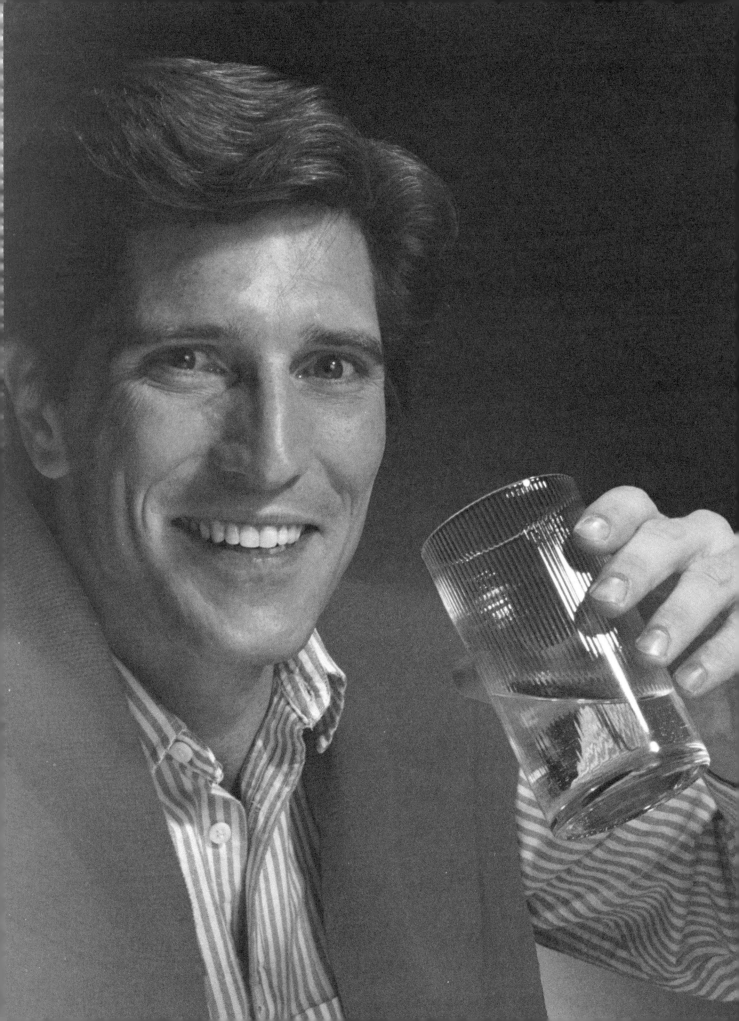

loaded with digestive enzymes. I could appreciate the advice Dr. Mervyn Hardinge, of Loma Linda University, gives in his health class: "The best time for water drinking is from one to two hours after meals and up to 10 to 15 minutes before meals.

Because we eliminate so much liquid through our kidneys, skin, lungs, and colon, we need to drink more than most of us do.

As I checked with my old physiology book I found that the digestive juices work best at normal body temperature, and if we drink ice water or other cold, (or very hot) beverages with our meals, this slows digestion until the stomach contents return to the right temperature. "Now that makes sense," I said to myself. "I should have thought of that before."

At work there was a drinking fountain just around the corner from my office door. I stopped there several times a day and mentally patted myself on the back for getting plenty of water.

Then another visitor, Joyce Hopp, health education secretary for the General Conference of Seventh-day Adventists, dropped in at the office. As she started to leave she spied the drinking fountain, bent her head down, and drank and drank. "She must be awfully thirsty," I decided.

But when she raised her head and wiped her mouth, she grinned and said, "Do you know how many swallows at a fountain it takes to equal a glass of water?"

"No, I never thought about it—How many?"

"Well, I did a little experimenting," she explained. "I took a glass to the drinking fountain, took a mouthful of water, and spit it into the glass. I did it again, again, and again. Guess how many it took."

"I don't know. I take a pretty big swig. Maybe six or eight."

"You ought to count it sometime. I tried it several times and found it runs between 15 and 20, depending on the size of your sip."

Now I keep a glass handy, fill it with water, and see to it that I drink several during the day. You know, you need at least six, and better eight, glasses in between meals.

Why do we need so much water?

Water is more than a thirst-quencher. It is the mainstream of your life—a solvent and dispersion medium for nutrients, electrolytes (minerals, mainly sodium and potassium), and waste products.

Let me tell you about my friend Henry.

When he knocked on my door, I assumed he had come on business, but he seemed in no hurry. He surprised me when he took a comfortable chair, leaned back, and rested his feet on a stool.

He drew a deep breath and sighed. "I'm so tired. I had a bad time on that trip to the convention last week.

"The water was awful. I just couldn't drink it. Then we got terrible news of a family tragedy. The shock threw me into a severe diarrhea attack that kept worsening until I was so dehydrated I collapsed to the floor—my mind so fuzzy and my mouth so dry I couldn't talk."

Fortunately, Henry's wife took over and called a doctor, who sent him by ambulance to the hospital.

"In the emergency room the doctor put fluids in a vein in my arm and made me drink as soon as I woke up.

"After four hours and replaced fluids, I

was OK," he told me. Then he confessed, "Since that episode I've been drinking water whether I like it or not."

Water makes up about 60 percent of your body weight because it is in all your tissues, inside the cells and around them. It is necessary for all of your body activities. Henry needed water to carry foodstuffs and other necessary things to every cell and to receive the wastes which his body produces. Some impurities gain entrance along with our food, drinks, and medicines, or are absorbed through the skin and inhaled in the air.

These impurities and other wastes must be dissolved and carried away in the blood and lymph, which are mostly water. If they are not, they cause you to become very tired, get sick, or even die. You need plenty of water to continually flush every cell with a rapidly circulating bath.[1]

Henry needed water to dissolve the wastes throughout his body and carry them to the skin, the lungs, and the kidneys, which got rid of them. An accumulation of wastes in your body can make you feel tired, weak, and maybe sleepy. Henry became so dopey he became unconscious, and so weak he fell to the floor.

A good drink or two can help your brain to be more alert.

Would you believe it? Even the gray matter of your brain is 85 percent water. About 93 percent of the blood is fluid so it can carry necessary substances to and from the cells.

The oxygen from the air could not get through the thin walls of the air sacs in the lungs if it was not first dissolved in a thin layer of fluid. And if the walls of the air sacs were perfectly dry, the carbon dioxide in the blood could not get out through the lungs.

Just think, you couldn't even blink your eyes if your eyes and the lids were really dry.

"While the glands that make the digestive juices secrete two to three gallons a day, they can't store this much water. So they make concentrated enzyme granules and then extract water from the bloodstream to add to them to make a juice of the right consistency, the way you make lemonade by adding water to a concentrate. When the digestive juice has served its purpose, the water is reabsorbed into the blood to be drawn out again to go another round, perhaps before you have finished your meal."[2]

When you work or play hard in summer, you notice the perspiration on your skin. This helps to control your temperature. Hikers, mountain climbers, and marathon runners find they tire less easily if they drink water along the way. Richard Kegley makes sure that someone has water waiting for him every so many miles along the route. This definitely delays fatigue and helps to prevent leg cramps.

Perhaps this is because water lubricates every part of your body and helps to protect your tissues from injury. It also makes your muscles, tendons, cartilage, and even your bones more flexible.

Yet, too much water can be harmful. One woman in our community became so weak that she fainted. Worried friends took her to the hospital, and when she gained consciousness, the doctor asked her a few questions. She revealed that the only thing she had done differently from usual was to drink a lot of water.

"How much?" the doctor asked.

"Oh, several gallons," she admitted. She

had read that most Americans don't drink enough water, and consequently she made sure she had plenty.

In her innocent ignorance she had drunk so much that she dangerously depleted her electrolytes (mineral salts)—important for regulating her heartbeat, kidney function, and mental alertness.

Would you know what to do if an accident happened to you? My little niece called me on the phone and cried, "Davie smashed his finger in the car door. He says it hurts awful bad, and it looks bluish. Mama's not here. What can I do?"

"Have him sit down," I told her, "while you get a pan of ice water. Have him keep his whole hand in it until it gets too cold for him to stand. Then let him take it out, but put it back into the ice water again until it either stops hurting or your mother gets home. Then if it isn't all right, she can call the doctor.

As a first-aid and home nursing instructor, I had learned that water often is the best thing to reach for in an emergency. If you sprain your ankle, place it in cold water immediately, and off and on during the first 24 hours. This helps to keep it from swelling and eases the pain.

Or if you burn yourself, you can submerge the injured area in cold water at once. Again, the cold water keeps it from hurting so bad, stops tissue destruction, and speeds up recovery. If the burn covers a large area or still hurts after an hour, you probably should check with your doctor to see if he suggests further treatment.

A hot footbath is an excellent means of relieving a headache, because it dilates the blood vessels in the your feet, and this draws the blood away from your head.

You probably love a refreshing shower or a relaxing soak in your tub. But a bath can do more than wash the dust and perspiration off your skin. It stimulates your circulation, which clears your brain, helps your digestion, and gets the white blood cells (germ fighters) into circulation, thus building up your resistance to disease.

An alternate hot and cold shower, ending with cold water and a vigorous rub to warm you, is an excellent "waker-upper" when you have a busy schedule ahead of you.

But suppose your hot and cold water is limited, like a soldier serving out on the battlefield. How could you manage?

Dr. Kenneth I. Burke, of the School of Allied Health Professions, Loma Linda University, tells his experience: "While in the U.S. Army in Germany, we spent extended periods of time in the winter 'in the field' with none of the niceties of civilization such as heated living quarters, hot water, etc. After about a week without a bath we would notice that we felt cold most of the time. If we would take a bath (cold water in a helmet), we would feel warm for a few days until gradually once again we would begin to feel cold all the time until we took another bath."

They hadn't imagined that the benefits of a cold bath would last that long.[3]

Perhaps scientists have more opportunity than most of us to recognize the blessings of God's handiworks. With this in mind, let's look at water from a chemist's viewpoint.

"Even an elementary school child can tell you that H_2O is the symbol for water, but few of us really understand how special it is.

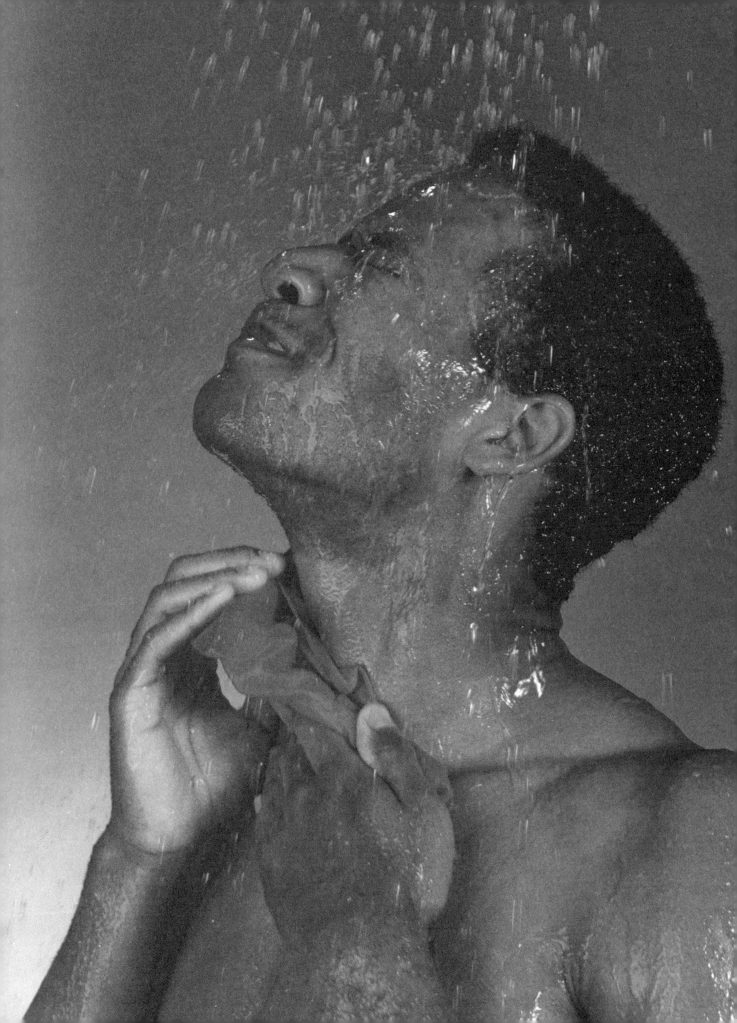

"Water appears to be a very simple substance made up of two parts of hydrogen and one part of oxygen, both of which are gases at ordinary temperature and rather difficult to liquify. However, God made it with most unusual characteristics—just right to meet our needs.

"Unlike other compounds that are considered liquid, it can be changed into a solid or gas without using extreme changes in temperature and pressure.

"When other liquids change to solids [freeze], they shrink or become more dense and sink to the bottom. But not water. Ice floats on top of the water instead of sinking to the bottom.

"Think what would happen if this were not true. Lakes and streams would be frozen solid with only a little cold water on the surface. Water plants and animals would be unable to survive.

"We often call water the universal solvent. Of course, it is not, for which we can be thankful. If it were, our houses, automobiles, and everything would dissolve, and we would be in a sad state of affairs. But water probably does dissolve a greater variety of substances than any other liquid. This makes it a most useful material, not only inside our bodies but all around us, for cleansing and for carrying nutrients to the roots of plants in the soil.

"Water has another strange characteristic. It requires more heat to raise the same amount of almost any other substance one degree temperature. Of course, this same amount of heat is given off when the water cools. This is why coastal areas have a milder climate than cities farther inland.

"This also means that fomentations [hot packs wrung from hot water] are very effective for transferring heat to an area of your body.

"It takes more calories of heat to melt an ounce of water than to melt an ounce of almost any other substance. So when you apply an ice pack to an injured foot, it cools it more efficiently than mere cold water. It also makes the blood and lymph vessels contract and reduce the swelling." [4]

Water has many uses that we seldom think about. We depend on it for manufacturing many things. For instance, it takes 650 gallons of water to make the steel for one bicycle, and more than 200 gallons to make the rubber in one car tire.

Beauty is another blessing of water. When did you last enjoy a colorful rainbow-crowned waterfall? The moonlight magic of a silver thaw? The dewdrop diamonds on your lawn? Can you remember when you last stretched out on the green grass and watched the ever-changing pictures in the clouds?

Wouldn't you just love to relax this afternoon beside a meandering river or a lazy little stream?

Water is another one of the truly great lifesavers.

---

[1] Mervyn Hardinge, *A Philosophy of Health*, p. 37.
[2] *Ibid.*, p. 38.
[3] Interview and correspondence with Kenneth I. Burke.
[4] Interview with Carl T. Jones, Dec. 20, 1987.

Lifesaver 8

TRUST

IN DIVINE POWER

"Could I pick you up and take you home after school this afternoon?" my friend Valerie called and asked me. The tension in her voice told me something was wrong.

"Yes. I think I'll have these papers graded by 4:15." I wondered what was on Val's mind. Had her marital problems taken a new twist? Was one of her three boys in trouble? Were her aged parents needing help again? Had her boss become even more unbearable?

I tried to hurry through my paper grading and preparations for the next day's classes, but my mind kept running away to Valerie.

When she arrived, I looked up to see deep worry lines in her forehead, and tears that she blinked away.

She drove to my house in silence and stopped the car in my driveway. She turned off the engine and turned to me. She sat there a moment longer, as if she didn't know what to say. Then she took a quick breath, as if ready to burst forth in a tragic report. But once again she bit her lip and sat in silence.

Finally she begged in a little cry for help, "Sometimes I just wish I had somebody to take my hand and say a little prayer for me."

Regretting that I had never done this for her, I quickly turned to our greatest Source of help.

I saw her fearful eyes turn in the direction of a passing car.

"I wondered if that was Bob," she said. "I don't want him to know I'm talking to you about it."

"Last night," she continued, "I was so scared I didn't know what to do. He was out late and came in really drunk. He kept looking out the window. Then he took his gun and laid it in a dresser drawer. He left the drawer open a little so he could grab the gun in an instant if he wanted to."

She was frightened for Bob's life — frightened that his befogged brain might even cause him to injure her or the boys.

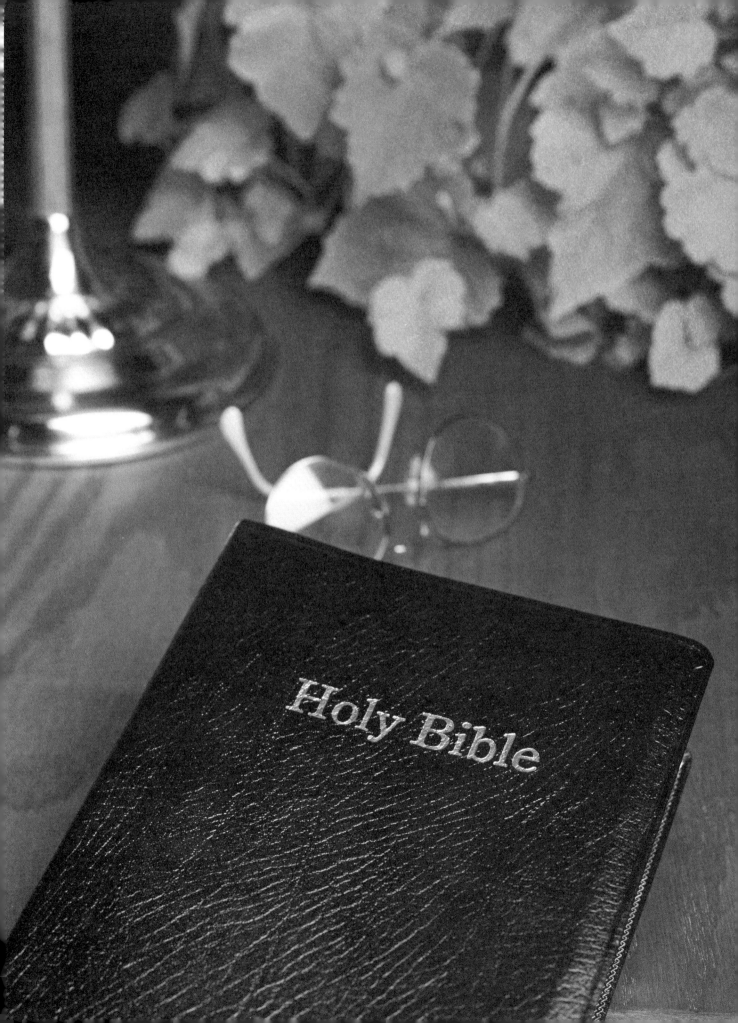

I watched the tired lines grow deeper in her face and heard the tension mount in her voice. I saw the tremor of her hands increase.

Things went from bad to worse, until the divorce was finalized.

Depression and anxiety are not restful. Stress is a monster that attacks every part of your body.

For a few months Val struggled to cope with her increased responsibilities. But she seemed to feel guilty for the broken home. And this guilt heightened her worry and stress.

> The mind is, by far, the most important aspect of the person. [1]

At the beginning of each school year Valerie had to have a physical examination. This time the doctor did not wear a smile

"I found a lump in your left breast," he told her. "Here's an order for a chest X-ray. I'll have the report next week. Come back on Tuesday."

I feared for Val because many studies show that anxiety, stress, and a loss like a divorce weaken a person's immune system. The defenses against disease break down.

"I'm scared," Val told me. "What if . . . what if . . .?

The seconds slowly ticked into minutes, hours, and days, until the week had gone.

I stayed near the phone the afternoon she was due to have news. Then she called. "The X-ray shows a tumor," she told me. "I had to have a bunch of blood tests, and next week I check into the hospital for surgery. . . . I don't know how extensive."

I went to the hospital and anxiously awaited the tragic report.

God gave her comfort and courage, but during those months of fright, grief, and guilt, her body had not been able to function well enough to fight off the lurking cancer. Our bodies work best when our minds are at peace, in a happy environment.

Now, not only do her children have to get along without a father, but without a mother as well.

> A merry heart maketh a cheerful countenance: but by sorrow of the heart the spirit is broken (Prov. 15:13).

God doesn't want us to be sick. This is the work of the enemy. God created Adam and Eve for fellowship. As long as they chose to maintain a close relationship with Him, they experienced a joyful existence. The happy experience of interacting with their Creator produced a positive reaction, enabling their perfect bodies and minds to function at the highest level of efficiency.

But when Adam and Eve broke this relationship, guilt, anxiety, grief, and other negative attitudes took over their thinking and controlled their body processes.

Doubtless, God desires to renew this healthful state of high immunity in us when he encourages us to develop the kind of relationships that will produce the exhilarating joyous laughter that promotes health and prolongs life.

Ecclesiastes 3:4 tells us there is "a time to laugh," and Proverbs 15:13 says, "A merry heart maketh a cheerful countenance: but by sorrow of the heart the spirit is broken."

Dr. Lee S. Berk, director of the psychoneuroimmunology laboratory, Department of Pathology, Loma Linda University, says, "We know that distress or experiences that bring out your negative emotions such as fear, grief, hate, and guilt are detrimental to your health because they lower your immunity to disease."

As in Valerie's case, it often has been noted that after a divorce, bereavement, or other great grief cancer seems to take hold more easily.

"Is it not possible, then," Berk reasons, "that some of the same substances may be decreased, or others increased, which would have a positive reaction and increase your immunity?"

Reseachers found that when you experience a positive emotional response such as joyous laughter, there is, indeed, a reduction in the negative hormones that would otherwise suppress the immune system. This experience, then, permits the immunity mechanism to function more effectively, protecting you from disease. [2,3]

In recognition of recent research on laughter and immunity, a number of hospitals across the country now have what they call the "Lively Room," the "Humor Room," or other laughter center. Doctors prescribe laughter as they would medication. And the results are encouraging. [4]

So what can you do to improve your family's health, their resistance to the germs that surround us? A good starting place might be to renew or enrich your relationship with your Creator. Let Him renew your courage, your hope, faith, and trust. This will lighten your burdens, fill your heart with joyous laughter, and put a song of thanksgiving on your lips.

A vibrant spirit of gratitude and praise can promote the health of your body and your soul.

Jay Lantry, an educator, returned to the United States after spending many years working in the Orient with people of 21 different languages.

He expected to earn a doctoral degree, but when the professors saw the scores on his entrance exam, they said, "We're sorry, but we can't let you into the doctoral program."

Being sponsored for the program by his church, Jay felt embarrassed and chagrined. How could he give up his plans and report his inabilities?

Overseas, Jay frequently had turned to prayer and faith to open closed doors. But he couldn't see how they could wipe out this barrier. The professors were adamant.

However, he had learned to trust God, and he remembered the promise, "Seek ye first the kingdom of God, and His righteousness and all these things shall be added unto you" (Matt. 6:33).

Could "all these things" include admission to the doctoral program? Jay wished it could. He knelt in submission and faith and promised, "Lord, if You will help me not only to be admitted, but to be a successful doctoral student, I will put Your Word first every day."

Then, armed with faith and new courage, Jay went back to the university and asked if the administration could possibly grant him provisional status and let him take classes for one semester.

At length, after listening to his request, they gave him permission to register for a few classes, although they didn't expect him ever to become a doctoral candidate. Jay went home challenged but determined to keep his promise to God. Every morning he rolled out of bed a whole hour earlier than he would need to do if he merely dressed, ate, and went to class. He religiously spent that hour in prayer and Bible study. Over and over he repeated, "Seek ye first the kingdom of God, and His righteousness, and I will add all these things unto you."

Jay says, "The first few weeks were horrid!" Unfortunately, in working for others, he had forgotten his own mother tongue. Were his professors right? Would he ever make it through the first semester, let alone three years, with passing grades?

How could he compete with classmates, who were masters of the English language? "My dictionary had a lot of use," he says.

Jay studied long hours. Every morning he continued to spend precious time in Bible study and fervent prayer. "And believe it or not," he told me, "by the end of the first semester my grades actually were far above the class average. The university administration waived my provisionary status and permitted me to enter the regular doctoral program.

"The second semester was a breeze," he declared, "because the Lord fulfilled His Word."

He went on to tell me that "never in the history of this university had the educational department had anyone complete a doctoral program in less than three years above the master's degree. Nevertheless, I finished everything for the doctorate in just a week or two less than 24 months, an all-time record for that school.

"Vocabulary is now one of my strong points," Dr. Lantry assured me, "and my mental capabilities have constantly expanded because I still put God first every morning. God never defaults on His word." [5]

Our heavenly Father has a thousand ways to provide for us, of which we know nothing. Those who accept the one principle of making the service of God supreme will find perplexities vanish, and a plain path before their feet. [6]

Our heavenly Father is no respecter of persons. He is waiting to do for you and me as much as He did for Dr. Lantry. We can trust Him to answer our prayers of faith in the manner best for us. He does not promise us a bed of roses in this sin-cursed land, but He does promise to be with us—and isn't that all we need?

Isn't our Saviour a great Lifesaver?

[1] Richard Neil, "The Answer," *Vibrant Life*, June 1987, p. 7.

[2] Interview with Dr. Lee S. Berk, Dec. 11, 1987.

[3] Lee S. Berk, D.H.Sc., M.P.H., F.A.C.S.M., "Modulation of Human Natural Killer Cells by Catecholamines," *Clinical Research*, 32, No. 1 (1984).

[4] Mike Schwartz, in Riverside (California) *Press Enterprise*, Nov. 9, 1987, Section C, pp. 1, 2.

[5] Don Stanley, "Hi! I'm Your Doctor. Have You Heard the One About—?" *The Sacramento Bee Magazine*, p.6.

[6] Ellen G. White, *The Desire of Ages* (Mountin View, Calif.: Pacific Press Pub. Assn., 1898), p. 330.

Chapter 9

LIFE AFTER...

Steve Canaday stuck his head through my office door. "Have you finished our grades yet?" he asked.

"Yes. I guess you want to know what you made."

"I sure do."

"Well, just let me check here. Your final grade is an A-minus. You really did well during the last half of the course."

"Thanks," he said. Then, pausing at the door, he turned with a big smile. "I'll tell you what I did.

"When I learned about the natural laws of health, I decided to practice them.

"When we studied the benefits of fresh air, sunshine, and exercise, I decided to go for a brisk walk or run every morning.

"When I realized how much sleep I need to do my best work, I made a program to include about eight hours a night.

"Of course, I never did use alcoholic drinks or cigarettes or coffee, so leaving them off was no problem.

"I did learn to drink more water, though. And when I learned how to balance my diet by using the four food groups, I chose my meals more carefully. When I learned the advantages of a lacto-ovovegetarian diet, I gave up eating meat. And when I realized what all that sugar was doing to me, I went to work to cut my dental bills.

"Then when I learned what a good breakfast would do for me, I ate like a king in the morning.

"I enjoy my Bible study more now, too." He gave me a big grin. "My grades have come up in my other courses, too."

I checked my record book, and sure enough, I discovered that on the first test Steve had gotten a C. On the second test he earned a B. On the third, an A–. On the fourth, an A. And on the final exam he had such a high A that it pulled his final grade up to an A-minus.

"Good for you, Steve," I said. "That kind of program can keep you right on top."

Steve is only one of thousands who have discovered that the NEWSTART program really works.

N utritious food
E xercise
W ater
S unlight
T emperate, drug-free living
A ir
R est
T rust in divine power.

Have you read about the lifestyle of Seventh-day Adventists and what it has done for them?

Seventh-day Adventists (SDAs) are a religious denomination of about 6 million. Most of them neither smoke tobacco nor drink alcoholic beverages.

In a 15-year study done by Roland L. Phillipps, Jan W. Kuzma, and Terry M. Lotz, Department of Biostatistics and Epidemiology, Loma Linda University, some very interesting facts came to light.

become a thoroughly good man is the best prescription for keeping a sound mind in a sound body."

Francis Bowen

The study revealed that "the risk of fatal cancer among SDA males is 53 percent of the risk among all United States White males of comparable age. For SDA females, the risk is 68 percent of that in all U.S. White females." Obviously, they are doing something right. Let us look a little further. When it comes to lung cancer, SDA men have only 17 percent of the risk that all White males in the U.S. have, and women have about 34 percent. This higher figure for women may be because not as many U.S. women smoke as do men.

ome folks seem to think religion is like a parachute—something to grab when an emergency occurs.

When we look at the record of deaths from *all* causes, the figures show that SDAs (both men and women) over 35 years of age have only 59 percent the risk of death that all U.S. Whites over 35 have.[1]

According to an article by Jane Brody in the New York *Times*, "over all, Adventists live seven years longer than the general American population, and for adherent Adventists, the average life expectancy is 12 years longer than the nation as a whole.

"Adventists have low rates, adjusted for age, of each of the 10 leading causes of death in this country, and especially low rates of such major afflictions as coronary heart disease and cancers of lung and bowel."

Heart disease deaths for Adventists "typically occur much later in life." [2]

Now that you see the real benefits of healthful living practices, you'll want to take hold of these Lifesavers and see where they'll take *you.*

HAPPY LIVING!

[1] Roland L. Phillipps, Jan W. Kuzma, and Terry M. Lotz, "Cancer Incidence in Defined Populations, New York, 1980," *Banbury Report 4* (Cold Spring Harbor Laboratory), pp. 93, 95, 96.
[2] Jane E. Brody, "Adventists Are Gold Mine for Research on Disease," New York *Times*, Nov. 11, 1986, p. 1.

APPENDIX

BREAKFAST RECIPES

Scrambled Tofu
(Tasty Egg Substitute)

1 lb. soft Tofu
¼ tsp. onion powder
¼ tsp. garlic salt, (optional)
2 tsp. soy sauce
1½ pkgs. Geo. Washington
    Golden Broth Mix
⅛ tsp. tumeric
    Few drops yellow coloring

Mash tofu and mix all ingredients. Cover with vented plastic. Cook in microwave on medium high for 2½ minutes. Stir and continue cooking for 1½ minutes. Stir and let stand one minute before serving.

Note: Instead of using the microwave, you can prepare this in a skillet or electric fry pan as you would scramble an egg.

Serve warm. Serves 4.

Granola
(fine textured)

4 cups quick oats
1 cup coconut
¼ cup wheat germ
½ cup chopped
    nuts
½ cup sunflower
    seeds
⅓ cup brown sugar
¼ cup honey
3 tbsp. corn oil
¾ tsp. salt
1½ tsp. vanilla
½ cup chopped
    dates or raisins

Mix first six ingredients in left column well. Mix honey, oil, salt, and vanilla and add to first mixture. Mix well. Microwave on High for 10 minutes or until oats are toasted, stirring every 4 minutes, and adding dates after 8 minutes. Sprinkle on cookie sheet to cool.

NOTE: You may use this granola for topping on cakes, puddings, or ice cream.

Makes 6 cups.

Read more

If you enjoyed reading the book in your hand, you might be interested in similar books offered by the Home Health Education Service. Turn this page for a brief description of the titles we publish for children as well as adults.

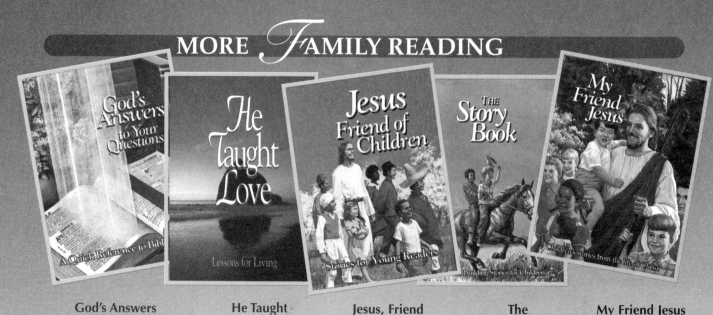
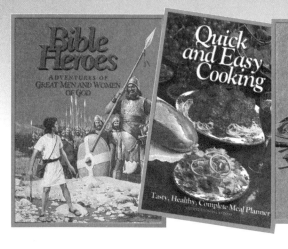
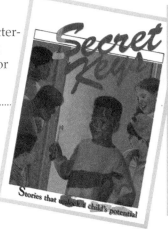
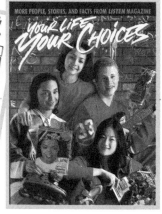